DIAGNOSTIC IMMUNOLOGY:
Current and Future Trends

CAP CONFERENCE / ASPEN 1978

PIERRE W. KEITGES, M.D., *Co-editor*

ROBERT M. NAKAMURA, M.D., *Co-editor*

Published by
COLLEGE OF AMERICAN PATHOLOGISTS
SKOKIE, ILLINOIS
1980

Library of Congress No. 79-54983
ISBN 0-930304-13-6

Table of Contents

PART IV. CELLULAR IMMUNITY

APPENDICES

INDEX

Preface

The College of American Pathologists has established a tradition through its Aspen Conferences dedicated to establishing a form for the discussion and review of new knowledge and problems concerning disciplines in laboratory medicine. In keeping with this spirit, it was decided in 1976 that an Aspen Conference on diagnostic immunology should be held as soon as possible. This conclusion stemmed primarily from the work of the Diagnostic Immunology Resource Committee of the CAP Council on Quality Assurance.

This group, through continued review of the CAP Survey data, became convinced of the needs for standards, reference methods and materials, and quality control procedures in the field of diagnostic immunology. It was apparent in laboratories throughout the country that there was an explosion of new knowledge in the area which resulted in a marked increase in the use of immunologic procedures in the hospital laboratory. However, much of the data generated by these tests did not have immediate apparent medical usefulness or clinical relevance, nor was there a means to monitor the accuracy and precision of these tests.

Given these problems, the Diagnostic Immunology Resource Committee was granted permission by the CAP Board of Governors to hold an Aspen Conference on diagnostic immunology in the fall of 1978. Forty experts in the field were invited to the conference. Immunologic assays in four areas were examined: immunoprecipitin techniques, immunofluorescence, enzyme labeled immunoassays, and cellular immunoassays. The current state of the art and future trends were analyzed in each area. The conference group made certain recommendations in regards to the development of reference methods, standards, and quality control procedures for various immunoassays. This volume is a review and summary not only of the deliberation of the conference, but its recommendations. The Aspen Conference participants would like to see their efforts stimulate the development of reference methods and materials, standards, and quality control procedures in the field of diagnostic immunology as it is applied in the modern hospital laboratory.

Co-directors P. W. Keitges, M.D., and R. M. Nakamura, M.D., wish to thank the participants in the conference for their dedication, initiative, and zeal in approaching the difficult laboratory problems in diagnostic immunology. In addition, the co-directors would like to thank CAP office personnel for their efficient and dedicated help in making the conference a success.

PIERRE W. KEITGES, M.D., *Co-editor*
ROBERT M. NAKAMURA, M.D., *Co-editor*
EDITORIAL BOARD, ASPEN CONFERENCE 1978
HAROLD E. BOWMAN, M.D.
SHARAD D. DEODHAR, M.D.

Recommendations of the College of American Pathologists Aspen Conference on Diagnostic Immunology

1. A task force should be established to develop a glossary for clinicians and clinical chemists using immunologic procedures.

2. The Diagnostic Immunology Resource Committee of the College of American Pathologists, the National Committee for Clinical Laboratory Standards, and the Center for Disease Control should work together cooperatively to develop a task force to seek solutions to the problems or questions raised at the conference.

3. A secondary control serum should be developed that would be immediately referable and transferable to the primary standard which is currently being developed and approved by the World Health Organization through the International Union of Immunological Societies. The secondary standard will initially be used to establish commonality of the interlaboratory comparisons in proficiency testing.

4. The College of American Pathologists will make available control sera for the 12 proteins of normal, high, and low values based on ranges of clinical relevance of that particular protein.

5. By some priority system, standard control sera characterized in several laboratories must be made available for each test system. The priorities can be established by those tests which are presently being introduced into the routine diagnostic laboratories.

6. Standardization of reference and assay procedures should be recognized as a primary need.

7. A task force should be assigned to determine that each reagent for reference methods has a procedure for standardization.

8. The most appropriate procedural approach in established standardized methodology should be selected from the ample existing information pertinent to all aspects of immunofluorescence.

9. Commercial producers should be involved much more intimately in efforts to establish and proliferate the standardized methodology selected.

10. Efforts should be continued to make reference reagents available as standards along with the various immunofluorescence systems.

11. A reference control system should be developed for the indirect IF ANA test. Sera from three systemic lupus erythematosus patients, or those with other systemic rheumatic diseases, in which the specific number of antibodies has been characterized and identified by the other specific immunologic tests should be made available. The three proposed reagents would be: (a) a titer of 1:160 or greater in the indirect IF ANA test, (b) a titer in the borderline range of 20-80, and (c) a normal sera in the range of less than 10 in the indirect IF ANA test.

12. A low-cost device should be developed for assessing the sensitivity of the fluorescent optical system.

13. Quality control procedures should be drafted for the indirect or the direct immunofluorescent test studies on biopsies and tissue procedures.

14. A checklist should be developed for the purpose of providing guidelines for laboratories that are interested in performing assays of this type.

15. A task force should be developed to provide some type of standard cell preparation.

Invited Participants and Guests
CAP Aspen Conference on Diagnostic Immunology

BARBARA P. BARNA, Ph.D.
Cleveland Clinic, Cleveland, Ohio

ERNST BEUTNER, Ph.D.
State University of New York, Buffalo, New York

HAROLD E. BOWMAN, M.D.
St. Mary's Hospital, Grand Rapids, Michigan

JOSEPH CAVALLARO, Ph.D.
Center for Disease Control, Atlanta, Georgia

LEO CAWLEY, M.D.
Wesley Medical Center, Wichita, Kansas

STEBENS CHANDOR, M.D.
State University of New York, Stoney Brook, New York

JERRY DANIELS, M.D.
University of Texas Medical Branch, Galveston, Texas

SHARAD DEODHAR, M.D.
Cleveland Clinic, Cleveland, Ohio

PAUL HORAN, Ph.D.
University of Rochester, Rochester, New York

PAUL E. HURTUBISE, Ph.D.
University of Cincinnati Medical Center, Cincinnati, Ohio

PIERRE W. KEITGES, M.D.
St. Joseph Hospital, Kansas City, Missouri

LARRY KILLINGSWORTH, Ph.D.
Sacred Heart Medical Center, Spokane, Washington

ROBERT NAKAMURA, M.D.
Scripps Clinic & Research Foundation, La Jolla, California

PAUL NAKANE, Ph.D.
University of Colorado, Denver, Colorado

DANIEL PALMER, Ph.D.
Center for Disease Control, Atlanta, Georgia

JOHN RIPPEY, M.D.
St. Lukes Hospital Laboratory, Kansas City, Missouri

ROBERT RITCHIE, M.D.
Maine Medical Center, Portland, Maine

STEPHAN RITZMANN, M.D.
Baylor Medical Center, Dallas, Texas

NOEL R. ROSE, M.D., Ph.D.
Wayne State University, Detroit, Michigan

HERBERT SOMMERS, M.D.
Northwestern Memorial Hospital, Chicago, Illinois

GEORGE C. SAUNDERS, V.M.D.
Los Alamos Scientific Laboratory, Los Alamos, New Mexico

JOHN SAVORY, Ph.D.
University of Virginia, Charlottesville, Virginia

RICHARD SCHNEIDER, Ph.D.
Syva Corporation, Palo Alto, California

H. J. TENOSO, Ph.D.
Organon, El Monte, California

KENNETH WALLS, Ph.D.
Center for Disease Control, Atlanta, Georgia

TAKESHI YOSHIDA, M.D.
University of Connecticut, Farmington, Connecticut

PART 1

DIAGNOSTIC IMMUNOLOGY

CHAPTER **I**

State of the Art of Immunoprecipitin Technics Using Agar Gels

L. P. CAWLEY, M.D.

Table of Contents

1. Introduction

Listed in Table I are the gel immuno-precipitin technics that have current utility for the clinical laboratory. The list is not complete, to be sure. Methods which are variations on the above list abound.

Each of the procedures consists of immunologic reactions in gels, substances that are optically clear but firm enough to support immunoprecipitin bands. The reaction may take several hours to days for completion. Those depending upon diffusion are driven by a process of spread under the force of molecular movement. The reaction with antibody or antigen occurs at collision points. In other gel technology, such as in the EID group, the reactants are forced together by electrical current. The end point may be evaluated in one of two ways—by visual inspection against an oblique light of the immuno-precipitin bands which appear white, or by photographic reproduction of the bands. More frequently now than before, the gels are processed for protein staining which improves the end point and leaves a permanent record for examination at leisure. In addition to these two approaches, isotope labeled antigen or antibodies have been used, with detection based on autoradiography. Recently, the use of enzyme labeled antibodies or antigens has resulted in patterns amplified by an enzyme stain.

2. Gel Diffusion (GD)

In Table II is a more detailed display of GD, EID, and IEP. Each of the three procedures listed in Table II is divisible into double and single systems. Double implies that both reactants move through the inert agarose gel during the diffusion. Antigen and antibody spread from their respective wells and react when the two diffusion fronts meet. Diffusion from a well is circular and the

Table I

PROCEDURES OF IMMUNOLOGIC
REACTIONS IN GELS

Technic	Abbreviation
Gel Diffusion	GD
Double	
Single (Radialimmunodiffusion)	(RID)
Electroimmunodiffusion	EID
Double (Counterelectrophoresis)	(CEP)
Single (Electroimmunoassay)	(EIA)
Immunoelectrophoresis	IEP
Double	
Single (two dimensional)	
Immune Complex Electrophoresis	ICE
Immunofixation Electrophoresis	IFE
Reverse Competitive Electro-immunodiffusion	RC EID
Backfire Electroimmunodiffusion	B EID

reactants become more dilute at the periphery since the periphery enlarges with diffusion. This dilution offers unlimited combination of antigen-antibody ratios, and the equivalent point is where the ratio produces a precipitate with all antigen being bound in the precipitate.

In single systems, in contrast to double, one reactant is relatively stationary, being placed in the gel while the other reactant (mobile phase) diffuses into the stationary phase. Usually the antibody is placed in the gel as in single GD, commonly known as radialimmunodiffusion (RID), and this is the direct mode used to quantitate antigen. Reverse single gel diffusion is the reverse, with antigen in the gel and antibody serving as the mobile phase. The direct single technic is most commonly performed in the laboratory for quantitation of immunoglobulins and other antigens. The concentration of specific antibody is measured by reverse single GD (reverse RID). The diffusion of either reactant into a contact gradiant of the other produces a circular zone of opacity whose diameter is related to the concentration of the diffus-

Table II

CLASSIFICATION OF IMMUNOLOGIC REACTIONS IN GELS

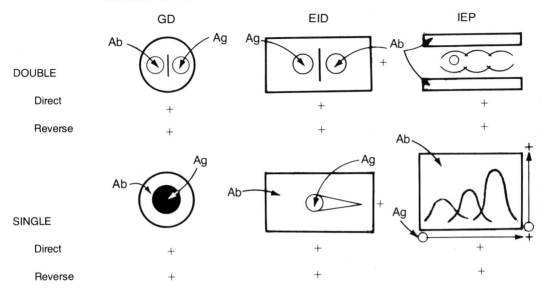

	GD	EID	IEP
DOUBLE			
Direct	+	+	+
Reverse	+	+	+
SINGLE			
Direct	+	+	+
Reverse	+	+	+

ing reactant. The concentration can be obtained by using a non-end point approach or by an end point system, the latter meaning the diffusion proceeds until no further growth of the precipitin rings occurs. Concentration obtained by either method gives results which are relatively uniform between procedures.

3. Electroimmunodiffusion (EID)

In the double system of EID, a direct current is incorporated into the system, which jokingly can be referred to as a "shocking Ouchterlony." The two reactants are forced toward, and into, each other by an electrical current. This procedure is also known as counterelectrophoresis (CEP). The most important aspect of this method is that the reactants are focused by the electrical field, resulting in greater sensitivity than that obtained by gel diffusion. As the molecules of each reactant are concentrated and driven toward each other, the number of possible unions or collisions is increased. For this reason, the method has enjoyed wide use in the laboratory,

as it is possible, by adjusting the buffer, the charge on the gel or on the reactant, to place the precipitin zone in a convenient position. The procedure is relatively rapid. It has found use in definition of antigens in spinal fluid, urine, exudates, and blood. To somewhat of a lesser extent than double GD, it is self-adjusting of ratio between antigen and antibody.

In single EID, the mobile reactant is propelled through the stationary, or immobile, reactant under the influence of an electrical current. In truth, the stationary phase is not truly immobilized; it moves by end-osmosis, although it may be made immobile by covalently linking the reactant to the agarose. The number of collisions between antibody and antigen is increased when antibody and antigen move toward each other. The precipitin zone continues to develop as long as the antigen is present. When the antigen becomes exhausted, the immunoprecipitin spike ceases to develop. The original technic was designated "monorockets" by Laurell and is an offshoot of work previously done by Dr. Ressler. Concentration of antigen in this technic is determined by recording the length of the spike, which is proportional to the log of the concentration. The procedure has enjoyed widespread utilization in Europe and, to a lesser extent, in the United States.

4. Immunoelectrophoresis (IEP)

IEP, as commonly used in the laboratory, is a double system in which both reactants move into an inert gel before coming in contact with each other. The first phase is electrophoresis and the second is the diffusion phase. Either antigen can be studied as in the direct approach, or antibody may be the point of interest in a reverse approach.

In the single system of IEP, commonly referred to as two-dimensional IEP, the first phase is electrophoresis as in the primary step to separate a reactant. In other words, the system can be direct or indirect; that is, it can be used to analyze antigen or antibody. In the case of the antigen, which is the most frequent use, it is referred to as the direct approach. The second phase of the technic involves

moving the separated proteins at right angles into a gel containing the second reactant, usually the antibody. The resultant pattern consists of multiple bell-shaped precipitin curves (Table II). The area under each curve is proportional to the concentration of the antigen. The technic has found wide use in Europe and limited use in the United States. From the diagram in Table II it can be seen that the overlapping immuno-precipitin bands produce a strikingly complex pattern.

5. Application of GD, EID, and IEP

Since the three approaches are the main tests of gel immunoprecipitin technics utilized in solution of clinical problems, a discussion of their use is in order. In Table III the various uses are stated, with each procedure recorded in the same format as Table II. Note that under each division, both the direct and reverse uses are recorded. Also note that the double systems of GD, EID, and

Table III

LABORATORY USES OF GD, EID AND IEP

	GD	EID	IEP
Detection and Separation			
Double	antibodies bacterial fungal auto	antibodies bacterial fungal auto	antibodies autoantibodies in IgA deficiency
	antigens bacterial fungal	antigens bacterial fungal	antigens monoclonal protein
Quantitation			
Single	antibodies quantitative	antibodies bacterial fungal auto	antibodies research
	antigens quantitative	antigens bacterial fungal	antigens monoclonal protein enzymes

IEP are all qualitative and are used either in the direct or reverse mode. What these procedures lack in sensitivity, they more than make up for in their power to resolve unusual mixtures of antigen and antibody. They require considerable expertise in interpretation. The double systems are under the general heading of detection and separation. It is of interest that many laboratory tests utilizing these principles frequently start with one or more of the double systems. Later, as an understanding of the system develops, the reagents may be improved to a point where a single system can be developed. Double gel diffusion systems are used first because little is known about the reagents in the early efforts to set up new procedures.

The single gel systems are designed for quantitation and depend on reagents that are more fully understood than in double systems. The latter frequently serve as the proving ground for each reagent to determine antibody specificity.

The three methods discussed—GD, EID, and IEP—are each divisible into two methods on the basis of single vs. double mode, giving a total of six methods, each of which in turn is divisible into two other modes, using the direct and the reverse approach, for a total of 12 separate technologies. With these procedures, most laboratories have been able to define many immunologic and infectious disorders. In some instances, however, these approaches are not up to the task.

Table IV is a short summary of diseases of immunologic nature where an alteration of some serum protein exists. In short, the procedures listed can resolve most all of the problems in Table IV except for clearly delineating minimonoclonal proteins in serum and cerebrospinal fluid, and detection of immune complexes, as listed under B, C, or D. It is true that two-dimensional IEP can characterize minimonoclonal

TABLE IV

LABORATORY USE OF IMMUNOLOGIC PRINCIPLES IN GELS ALTERED CHANGE IN SERUM PROTEINS

A. Malignant plasma cell clone
   Monoclonal protein, including Bence Jones protein
   Alteration of Ig balance

B. Nonmalignant plasma clonal proliferation
   Minimonoclonal protein

C. Autoimmune disease
   Polyclonal gammopathy with minimonoclonal production
   Autoantibodies

D. Immune complex disease
   Activation of C and miniband formation

E. Deficiencies acquired/congenital
   Ig
   Alpha$_1$ antitrypsin
   G6PD

F. Binding proteins
   Lipoproteins

G. Chronic or acute inflammation
   Acute phase proteins with and without polyclonal gammopathy

proteins and that IEP also can. However, two-dimensional IEP is difficult and time consuming, while IEP often fails because of poor resolution.

6. Additional Technics of Immunoprecipitin Reactions in Gels

The additional procedures listed in Table V consist of four which have properties that are unique and extend the power of immunogel reactions. Some of these can answer the questions raised in B, C, or D of Table IV. The presence of minimonoclonal proteins in cerebrospinal fluid, serum, or urine represents one of the observations currently being made in laboratories utilizing high resolution agarose gel electrophoresis. Protein zones of restricted electrophoretic mobility often bear on a significant disease, and in many instances, identification and characterization of these minimonoclonal proteins are important

Table V

FOUR IMMUNOGEL TECHNICS FOR DETECTION OF ANTIGEN/ANTIBODY

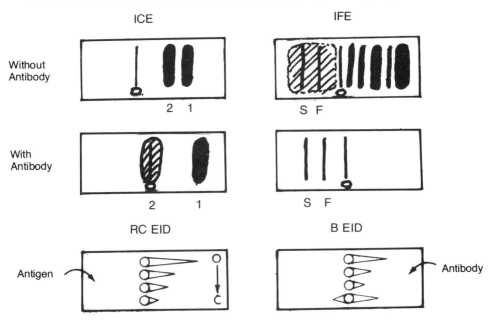

to the patient. The term minimonoclonal protein implies a small concise band which is just visible in the electrophoretic pattern. Sometimes these bands are multiple and only become noticeable after immunofixation electrophoresis (IFE). The technic of IFE is superior to IEP for the identification of minimonoclonal proteins. It is an additive procedure. Antisera is applied directly to the surface of the gel after electrophoresis, diffuses into the gel, and fixes the desired antigen (or antibody in the reverse mode). All uncombined proteins are removed and the immunofixed components are stained for protein. An antibody labeled with an isotope or with an enzyme increases the sensitivity manyfold. Because the antisera diffuses for such a short distance before reaching the antigen, the minimonoclonal proteins become fixed in the gel and remain fixed without diffusing, thereby preserving the separation afforded by high resolution agarose electrophoresis. In immunoelectrophoresis, the diffuse phase causes a blurring of bands and loss of

resolution. The procedure is most often used as a multiple channel system with a monospecific antibody in each channel. For example, antibodies to IgG, IgA, and IgM and kappa and lambda constitute a five-channel system.

The detection of immune complexes, which answers question C in Table V, can best be handled by a technic known as "backfire rocketry." It involves the concept of using basic EID with anti-C3 (also anti-C4 and anti-C3PA). During EID, the complement moves toward its proper electrophoretically determined mobility point, and in the course of that, combines with antibody and forms a precipitin spike referred to as a rocket. If complement has become bound with an antigen-antibody complex, its mobility is altered, and this altered mobility is frequently on the reverse side of the origin. A discharge or backfire to the cathodic side of any rocket is adjudged to be an immune complex. These patterns have been shown to be related to diseases associated with immune complex disease.

7. Immune Complex Electrophoresis (ICE)

This procedure is of interest and has utility in identifying certain isoenzymes. An antibody to placental alkaline phosphatase, when mixed with a serum known to contain multiple alkaline phosphatase isoenzymes just before the electrophoretic phase, will form an immune complex which remains at the point of origin. After the electrophoresis, a histochemical stain is performed for alkaline phosphatase. As shown in Table V, if there are two components—one and two—the complex formed by the antibody and antigen reaction remains at the origin while the uninvolved isoenzyme band moves to its customary position. This has been applied against alkaline phosphatase isoenzymes, CPK isoenzyme, and hemoglobin variants with success.

8. Reverse Competitive EID (RC EID)

For quantitation with enzyme labeled antibodies, this procedure approaches RIA in sensitivity. The gel contains antigen; for example, IgG and the antisera bearing the enzyme label is anti-IgG. Since this is a reverse technic, the labeled antibody moves into the gel and reacts with the antigen, forming a rocket. By adding serum IgG or standards of IgG to the labeled antibody, it is possible to inhibit the mobility of the labeled antibody, causing some of it to remain at the point of application as a complex. The reverse competitive EID method generates calibration curves like those of RIA. The approach is highly sensitive and simple.

9. References

Afonso, E. (1964). *Clin Chim Acta* **10**, 114

Alper, C. A. (1971). *In* "Progress in Immunology" (Amos, B., ed.) p. 609, Academic Press, New York

Alper, C. A. and Johnson, A. M. (1969). *Vox Sang* **17**, 445

Arnaud, P., Wilson, G. B., Koistinen, J. and Fudenberg, H. H. (1977). *J Immunol Meth* **16**, 221

Arquembourg, P. C. (1975). *In* "Immunoelectrophoresis—Theory, Methods, Identification, Interpretation," 2nd Edition, S. Krager, Basel

Axelsen, N. H., Kroll, J. and Weeke, B. (1973). *In* "A Manual of Quantitative Immunoelectrophoresis. Methods and Applications," Universitetsforlaget, Oslo

Bussard, A. (1959). *Biochim Biophys Acta* **34**, 258

Carrel, S., Theilkaes, L., Skvaril, S. and Barandun, S. (1969). *J. Chromatog* **45**, 483

Cawley, L. P. (1969). *In* "Electrophoresis and Immunoelectrophoresis," Little, Brown & Co., Boston

Cawley, L. P. (1974). *In* "Enzymology in the Practice of Laboratory Medicine" (Blume, P., and Freier, E. F., eds.) pp. 323-349, Academic Press, Inc., New York and London

Cawley, L. P. (1975). *In* "Proceedings of the Pine Mountain Conference of Diagnostic Immunochemistry," American Association for Clinical Chemistry

Cawley, L. P. and Eberhardt, L. (1962). *Amer J Clin Path* **38**, 539

Cawley, L. P., Minard, B. J. and Chelle, C. (1976). *Clin Chem* **22**, 1201

Cawley, L. P., Minard, B. J. and Chelle, C. (In press). *Amer J Clin Path*

Cawley, L. P., Minard, B. J. and Grohs, H. K. (In press). *Clin Chem*

Cawley, L. P., Minard, B. and Penn, G. M. (1978). "Electrophoresis and immunochemical reactions in gels," 2nd Edition, Education Products Div., American Society of Clinical Pathologists, Chicago

Cawley, L. P., Minard, B. J., Tourtellotte, W. W., Ma, B. I. and Chelle, C. (1976). *Clin Chem* **22**, 1262

Cejka, J. and Kithier, K. (1976). *Immunochem* **13**, 629

Chang, C. H. and Inglis, N. R. (1975). *Clin Chim Acta* **65**, 91

Crowle, A. J. (1973). *In* "Immunodiffusion," 2nd Edition, Academic Press, New York

Drysdale, J. W. and Singer, R. M. (1974). *Cancer Res* **34**, 3352

Fahey, J. L. and McKelvey, E. M. (1965). *J Immunol* **94**, 84-90

Frohlich, J., Cawley, L. P. and Campbell, D. J. (1976). *Ann R Coll Physicians Surg Can* **9**, 54

Gocke, D. J. and Howe, C. (1970). *J Immunol* **104**, 1031

Grabar, P. and Williams, C. A., Jr. (1953). *Biochim Biophys Acta* **10**, 193-194

Grassman, W. and Hubner, L. (1953). *Naturwiss* **40**, 272

Keck, K., Gorssberg, A. L. and Pressman, D. (1973). *Eur J Immunol* **3**, 99

Kohn, J. (1970). *J Clin Path* **23**, 733

Johnson, A. M. (1976). *J Lab Clin Med* **87**, 152

Laurell, C. B. (1965). *Anal Biochem* **10**, 358

Laurell, C. B. (1966). *Anal Biochem* **15**, 45

Laurell, C. B. (ed.) (1972). *Scan J Clin Lab Invest* **29**, suppl. 124

Makonkawkeyoon, S. and Haque, R. (1970). *Anal Biochem* **36**, 422

Mancini, G, Carbonara, A. O. and Heremans, J. F. (1965). *Immunochem* **2**, 235

Merrill, D., Hartley, T. F. and Claman, H. N. (1967). *J Lab Clin Med* **69**, 1, 151-159

Minard, B. J. and Cawley, L. P. (1974). *Amer J Clin Path* **62**, 306

Nakamura, S. and Ueta, T. (1958). *Nature* **182**, 875

Ouchterlony, O. (1949). *Acta Path Microbiol Scand* **26**, 507

Oudin, J. (1946). *C R Acad Sci* **222**, 115

Ressler, N. (1960). *Clin Chim Acta* **5**, 795

Ritchie, R. F. and Smith, R. (1976). *Clin Chem* **22**, 497

Ritchie, R. F. and Smith, R. (1976). *Clin Chem* **22**, 1982

Van Lente, F. and Galen, R. S. (In press). *Clin Chim Acta*

Weeke, B. (1970). *Scand J Clin Lab Invest* **25**, 161-163

Zeineh, R. A., Mbawa, E. H., Pillary, V. K. G., Fiorella, B. J. and Dunea, G. (1973). *J Lab Clin Med* **82**, 326

Zydeck, F. A., Muirhead, E. E. and Schneider, H. (1965). *Nature* **205**, 189-190

CHAPTER ▐▐

State of the Art of Nephelometry

J. SAVORY, Ph.D.

Table of Contents

1. Introduction

Quantitative immunochemistry was introduced by Heidelberger and Kendall (1929; 1932; Heidelberger *et al*, 1936) in their classic work on the precipitin reaction between Type III pneumococcus polysaccharide and its homologous antibody. These investigations provided the theoretical basis for the development of a series of analytical methods for the determination of specific proteins. The technique was first applied in a clinical situation by Goettsch and Kendall (1935) for the estimation of albumin and globulin in human serum. Subsequent studies involved estimation of protein in other body fluids of interest in a variety of diseases (Goettsch and Reeves, 1936; Kendall, 1938; Kabat *et al*, 1948), and the diagnostic value of protein measurements became well established.

Beginning in 1946, several procedures were developed which were based on the migration of the antigen and an antibody molecule through an agar gel matrix. The simple diffusion system of Oudin (1946) was the first to employ this principle; the method can be both precise and sensitive and is still a useful tool for measurement of proteins in dilute solutions.

The technique of immunoelectrophoresis, described by Grabar and Williams in 1953 and modified by Scheidegger in 1955, allows for examination of complex protein mixtures without prior purification steps. The semiquantitative results obtained from immunoelectrophoresis have limited clinical application except in the classification of monoclonal gammopathies of various types and in deficiencies of certain serum proteins (Grabar and Burtin, 1964; Clarke and Freeman, 1968).

The development of radial immunodiffusion by Mancini, Carbonara, and Heremans (1965) and others (Fahey and McKelvey, 1965; Lou and Shanbron, 1967) brought about a new era in the immunochemical measurement of proteins in biological fluids. This method gained a wide popularity not attained by those described previously, and it has retained that popularity into the present. The commercial availability of radial immunodiffusion "kits" has facilitated the use of this technique for the quantitation of numerous proteins of clinical importance. Radial immunodiffusion is deficient, however, in that it is imprecise, time consuming, and lacks the sensitivity required to detect most proteins in unconcentrated cerebrospinal fluid and urine. These deficiencies have prompted the development of alternate procedures which are described below.

Determination of the concentration of proteins by electrophoresis into antibody-containing agarose gel was introduced by Laurell (1965; 1966) at about the same time Mancini *et al* (1965) published their work on radial immunodiffusion. The technique, known as electroimmunodiffusion, differs from radial immunodiffusion in that an electrical field is employed to force migration of the antigen into the gel. In some cases, as little as $0.1\mu g$ of antigen can be detected. Many human proteins have been measured by electroimmunodiffusion in a few specialized laboratories, but the method has not attained widespread use since numerous technical details must be mastered in order to obtain acceptable results.

As an alternative to the analysis of proteins through their migration in a gel, the precipitin reaction may be quantitated by optical measurements of aqueous solutions. In 1947, Boyden and co-workers (1947) introduced the concept that precipitin curves could be characterized through the measurement of the turbidity which developed in mixtures of antigen and antibody. Their studies showed that turbidity values correlated closely with the actual amounts of precipitate formed in the immunochemical reaction.

This approach was not applied to clinical measurements until Schultze and Schwick (1959) published their turbidimetric methods for determining several plasma proteins. Ritchie (1967) later improved this technique so that very small amounts of sample and antiserum could be utilized, and measurements could be made on a standard spectrophotometer. The results obtained proved to be reliable and precise, and it was suggested that the method would be useful for the estimation of immunoglobulins in human serum. Alper et al (1969) also utilized turbidimetric analysis in studies on the inherited deficiency of the third component of complement (C3), but did not discuss details of the procedure. The use of turbidimetric analysis in immunochemistry has been discussed by Leone (1971) and Li and Williams (1971); their studies showed that turbidimetry could be useful in determining the quality and quantity of specific antigens in the presence of other antigens or contaminants of the same type.

Interest in quantitation of immunochemical reactions by optical measurements of aqueous solutions has increased in the past few years. The need to automate diagnostic immunochemical tests has resulted in several procedures based on nephelometric measurements of immune complexes. Nephelometric, or light-scattering, procedures usually detect light at a 90° angle to the incident light, and can be performed on slightly modified filter fluorometers; however, recently other angles of detection have been employed. These nephelometric techniques are capable of greater sensitivity than those employing turbidimetry and are easily automated in either discrete sample or continuous flow systems.

Eckman et al (1970) reported the first automated immunoprecipitin technique for use with modules of the Technicon Corporation Autoanalyzer. Existing components of the Autoanalyzer system were used to dilute serum samples, provide mixing with antiserum, and make light-scattering measurements for the determination of human transferrin. Analyses were performed at a rate of 60 per hour with good precision and accuracy. This initial study provided the impetus for several other groups of investigators to develop additional manual and automated procedures for the analysis of proteins in human serum (Killingsworth et al, 1971; Killingsworth and Savory, 1971; Larson et al, 1971; Alper, 1971; Wegfahrt et al, 1971; Killingsworth and Savory, 1972; Savory and Killingsworth, 1973), cerebrospinal fluid (Ritchie and Graves, 1971; Savory et al, 1972; Killingsworth and Savory, 1973b), and urine.

2. Principle

The specific protein (antigen) in the body fluid reacts with antibody in a specific antiserum to form antigen-antibody (Ag/Ab) complexes which can be detected by light-scattering techniques. The Ag/Ab reaction can be characterized by a precipitin-like curve, such as that shown in Figure 1, which reflects the change in particle size and number caused by increasing Ag/Ab ratios. In this specific example, a series of serum samples containing IgG at concentrations ranging from 500-3000 mg/dl was diluted 1:700 with dust-free physiologic saline. One part of diluted sample was mixed with one part of diluted goat anti-human IgG, and after 40 minutes at room temperature, Ag/Ab complex formation achieved an equilibrium state and light-scattering measurements were made in fluorometer with identical excitation and emission wavelengths (360nm).

The first section of the precipitin curve (Figure 1), where light-scattering intensity increases with concentration of IgG, is termed the antibody excess zone.

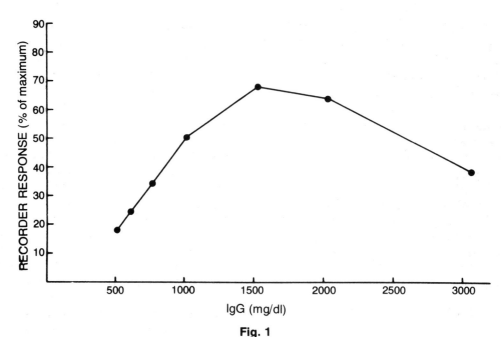

Fig. 1

Precipitin curve for the IgG/anti-IgG complex. (Reprinted by permission of Clinical Chemistry, *18*, 337 (1972).

There is an equivalence zone at the apex of the curve and an antigen excess zone where intensity decreases with increasing IgG concentration. Qualitative data dealing with all zones of the precipitin curve have revealed that Ag/Ab complex size and/or concentration increases through antibody excess, reaching a limiting value at equivalence and then dropping in antigen excess. The pattern is thought to be a function of the antigen to antibody site ratio. As the number of antigen sites increases, a greater number of complexes are formed in antibody excess until site equivalence is reached and a limiting particle size and concentration result. The further addition of antigen results in smaller complexes due to the excess of antigenic sites, and reduced cross linking between aggregates occurs.

3. Factors Affecting Light-Scattering Procedures

A. Antiserum

Most laboratories rely on antiserum from commercial sources. In all cases, the monospecificity of the antiserum should be confirmed by observation of a single precipitin arc on immunoelectrophoresis against whole human serum. The degree of dilution of the antiserum prior to the immunochemical reaction depends on the avidity of the antiserum. Thus, a precipitin curve should be constructed with each new batch of antiserum, and the dilution adjusted to give adequate sensitivity and a broad range of antigen concentrations in the antibody excess zone.

B. Reagent Preparation

Exogenous particulate matter such as dust causes serious interferences in light-scattering measurements. All diluent buffer solutions and diluted antisera must be filtered prior to use. Filters with an average pore size of $0.22\mu m$ provide satisfactory results.

C. Wavelength

For non-polarized incident light, Rayleigh's law states that the intensity of scattered light is inversely proportional to the fourth power of the wavelength; for this reason, a wavelength of 360nm is used on most commercially-available instruments. Higher wavelengths may be used if the source possesses greater intensity. Usually, adequate sensitivity can be achieved up to 650nm provided a high intensity source is used. The limiting feature is not the actual total intensity of light scattered, but the difference in intensity of the sample vs. the sample blank. Most biological fluids possess high background light-scattering, and reaction conditions must be adjusted so that the immunochemical reaction gives considerably more scatter than the background.

D. Angular Variation

In the past, virtually all light-scattering photometers now used for measurements of proteins by immunochemical methods measured light-scattering at 90°; however, it has been known for many years that increases in scattering intensity can be obtained at angles less than 90° when large particles are considered. According to Rayleigh, the intensity of scatter from a particle, which is small relative to the wavelength, should be distributed symmetrically about an axis which is at right angles to the incident beam. However, for particles whose dimension is comparable to the wavelength of light used for analysis, destructive interference of the light scattered from individual elements can occur, resulting in a decrease in total scattering measured. Phase difference between scattered radiation, which causes the destructive interference, is reduced as the angle of observation approaches zero, resulting in an asymmetrical scattering envelope and significant angular dependence. Shown in Figure 2 are angular dependent scattering intensity measurements for a particular Ag/Ab ratio using the IgM/anti-IgM reac-

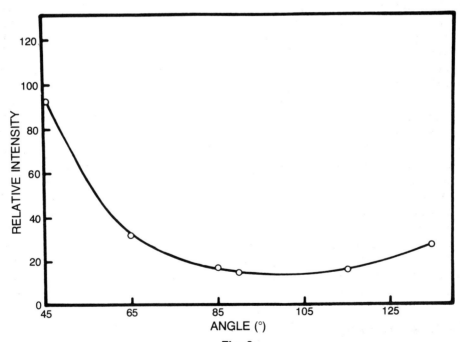

Fig. 2
LIGHT SCATTERING AS A FUNCTION OF ANGLE
IgM/ANTI-IgM   [IgM] = 1.30 μg/ml
Change in light-scattering intensity as a function of angle for IgM/anti-IgM reaction products.
(Reprinted by permission of Clinical Chemistry, 21, 1738, (1975).

tion as an example. It is obvious that the scattering measured is least intense at 90° and markedly increased in intensity at smaller angles. If the particles were homogeneous with respect to size and shape, a series of light-scattering maxima and minima should have been observed as a function of the angle of observation, according to the Mie theory. However, no intensity maxima or minima are observed as a function of angle, indicating that the complex population is a polydisperse system with respect to size.

E. Effects of Temperature, pH, and Urea

Using an IgG/anti-IgG model system, the effects of temperature, pH and a variety of urea concentrations have been studied (Killingsworth and Savory, 1973a), and it was demonstrated that temperature and pH, if controlled within reasonable limits, cause minimal variations in the Ag/Ab reaction. Urea, which is present in body fluids, sometimes at relatively high levels, has an appreciable effect of inhibiting the reaction. Thus, for urine analysis, attention must be paid to the urea concentration of the final reaction mixture in order to ensure that pronounced inhibition of the Ag/Ab reaction does not occur.

F. Effects of Ions in the Reaction Medium

Using the IgG/anti-IgG reaction as an example, it can be demonstrated that this reaction is quite sensitive to changes in ionic strength. A decrease in the sodium chloride concentration results in a profound enhancement of the reaction rate. Apparent molecular weight and radius of gyration determined by light-scattering (Buffone *et al*, 1975) in the presence and absence of sodium chloride has demonstrated that the complex dimension is apparently constant, while the average molecular weight appears to be decreased in the solution of higher ionic strength. It appears that the effect of sodium chloride is to slow the reaction rate so that fewer complexes are produced within the time frame of the analysis, while the character of the complexes remains unaffected. These results are consistent with the theory that negatively-charged ions, such as Cl-, compete with the negatively-charged binding sites on the antigens for binding sites on the antibody. A reduced rate and an unaltered product would be expected.

The ion character also produces significant differences in the observed kinetics of the reaction. The rate of increase in light-scattering measured at 90° is decreased by certain neutral salts. The efficacy of reduction is in the order $NO_3^- >$ $Br^- > F^-$ (with the same cation) using the IgG/anti-IgG systems (Killingsworth and Savory, 1973a).

G. Effect of Polymers and Proteins

Water-soluble straight-chain polymers have been used to enhance the signal for the Ag/Ab reaction, thereby increasing sensitivity and reducing analysis time (Hellsing, 1972).

Studying the IgG and anti-IgG system with polyethylene glycol (PEG, molecular weight 6000) in the reaction medium, one notes a lag period in the rate of change in light-scattering during the first 5 s of the reaction. After the initial 5 s, however, the rate increases markedly and the reaction proceeds much more rapidly in PEG (40 g/liter) plus phosphate-buffered physiological saline than in phosphate-buffered physiological saline alone.

4. Instrumentation

The original manual procedures (Killingsworth and Savory, 1972; Savory and Killingsworth, 1973) involved dilutions made with an automated pipetting device, with light-scattering measurements being carried out on either a filter or grating spectrophotofluorometer. Because of the relative lack of dependence of the measurement on the wavelength of the incident light, filter instruments were found to be quite satisfactory. Most of the early instruments used 90° light-scattering on a conventional spectrophotofluorometer. Recently, an instrument dedicated to nephelometry has been introduced where 90° light-scattering is measured, but the incident light appears through the bottom of the cuvette (Kallestad Laboratories Inc., Chaska, Minn. 55318).

The introduction of near forward light-scattering with laser light sources (Buffone et al, 1974; Buffone et al, 1974) has led to the development of two commercial laser nephelometers. The lasers employed are inexpensive helium neon lasers which emit light at a wavelength of 632.8nm. The advantages of using lasers are the intensity of the light, simplified optical system, and adaptability to forward light-scattering measurements. The Hyland Laser Nephelometer (Hyland, Division of Travenol Laboratories, Inc., Costa Mesa, Calif. 92626) uses an optical configuration with an angle of measurement of 31°. The Behring Laser Nephelometer (Behring Diagnostics, American Hoechst Corp., Somerville, N.J., 08876) uses a dark field similar to the first near forward light-scattering system developed in the author's laboratory which is described later. The angle of measurement with the Behring instrument is from 5°-12°.

Many tedious dilutions are required for manual systems, and computation of results is time consuming. For these reasons, the tendency today is to use some type of semi-automatic dilutor and to integrate the nephelometer with a microprocessor for calculation of results.

A manual nephelometer which performs analyses using kinetic measurements has recently become available from Beckman Instrument Company (Fullerton, Calif. 92634). This rate nephelometer uses a tungsten/iodine light source, and scattered light is detected at a 70° angle. The instrument measures the rate of increase in intensity of scattered light, and a microprocessor converts the peak rate into concentration. The microprocessor is programmed by a card which carries information on a specific test for curve fitting, analysis time, antigen excess detection criteria, analyte identification, and instrument gain.

The most widely-used automated approaches to nephelometry have been with the centrifugal analyzer and with continuous flow systems. The first description of the use of a centrifugal analyzer for the measurement of specific proteins was by Tiffany et al (1974). These workers used a miniature centrifugal analyzer modified for fluorescence and light-scattering measurements, the latter being carried out at 410nm. The cuvettes held 120 to 150μl of reaction mixture, with mixing of reactants being accomplished at a Y-junction following acceleration of the rotor, with rapid acceleration and deceleration used to ensure complete mixing. Light-scattering measurements could be made approximately 6 s after constant speed was attained. Computer control of the instrument enabled readings of light-scatter to be made at any predetermined time.

The major problems with the instrument used by Tiffany et al (1974) are its lack of availability on the commercial market and, even assuming access to the miniature centrifugal analyzer, the extensive modifications necessary for 90° light-scattering. In order to adapt kinetic methods to an available commercial centrifugal analyzer, Buffone et al (1974; 1974; 1975; 1975; 1975) modified existing equipment to measure near 0° angle light-scattering. This approach involved a simple modification of the optical system of a commercial centrifugal analyzer

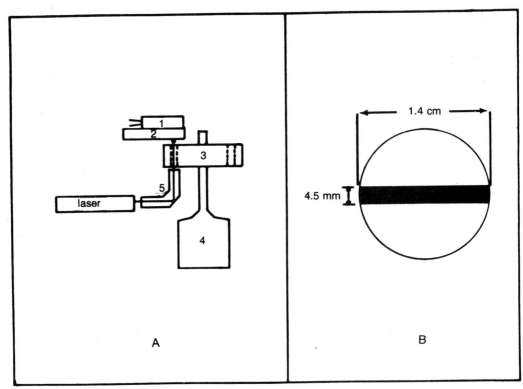

Fig. 3

(A) Schematic diagram of laser-modified parallel fast analyzer: 1, photodiode; 2, interference filter wheel; 3, rotor assembly; 4, centrifuge motor; 5, shielded optical path containing mirror.

(B) Dark field design used in present modification of parallel fast analyzer system.

(Reprinted by permission of Analytical Chemistry, 46, 2047, (1974).

equipped for conventional visible and ultraviolet spectroscopic analysis, with changes being made to allow only scattered light to reach the detector while blocking out all light coming directly from the source. An Aminco Rotochem II centrifugal analyzer (American Instrument Company, Silver Spring, Maryland 20910) was modified with the following three basic changes: replacement of the tungsten-halogen lamp with a helium-neon gas laser (alignment of the laser is most easily accomplished with the rotor removed from the instrument); removal of both lenses located in the optical path; and placement of a dark field between the cuvettes and the detector.

A schematic diagram of the apparatus and dark field disc is shown in Figures 3A and 3B. The optical system consisted of a helium-neon gas laser (Spectra Physics, Mountain View, Calif. 94040, Model 155, 632.8nm) which has a peak power output of 0.5mW and is, therefore, a relatively safe laser to use on a routine basis. Long-term stability is rated at 5% of output power drift. A constant-voltage transformer (Sola Electric, Elk Grove Village, Ill. 60007) was used to reduce variation in line voltage reaching the laser. The laser beam was directed through the cuvettes to the detector by means of a mirror positioned at a 45° angle to the incident beam (Figure 3A). The primary reason for using the laser was to minimize the modification of the optical system. The cuvette assembly, made up of 15 cuvettes, was formed from a stainless steel heat pack sandwiched between two pieces of quartz. A dark field was interposed between the cuvettes and the detector to block out light coming directly from the source, thereby allowing only scattered light to reach the detector. The dark field was made up of a circular piece of quartz 1.4cm in diameter and 1.0mm thick (Figure 3B). Optical black paint was used to block out an area 4.5mm wide and 2.5cm long across the center of the quartz disc. The detector was a custom photodiode with a radiometrically-determined optimum range of 250 to 620nm. The signal was passed directly from the photodiode through a band-pass-limited amplifier and was processed by an analog-digital converter. Data accumulation and averaging were controlled by a PDP/8M minicomputer (Digital Equipment Corp., Maynard, Mass. 01754). A single absorbance or transmittance reading for a cuvette was obtained by averaging the digital signal over eight consecutive revolutions of the rotor to improve the signal-to-noise characteristics. Data was processed by the computer and then displayed by a high-speed (30 characters/s) printer terminal.

The concept of a dark field and focused source beam is currently in use in the field of microscopy. The need to use lenses to focus the output from a conventional incandescent source can be eliminated if a laser source is employed. The laser source provides a highly collimated and intense beam allowing dark field size to remain at a minimum. The combination of a highly collimated source beam and minimum field size allows maximization of the signal-to-noise ratio.

Several dark field designs were tested. A relatively high signal-to-noise ratio should be obtainable with a small circular field; however, the use of this type of field resulted in an asymmetrical signal, with large spikes being seen on one edge of the signal from each cuvette. The asymmetrical signals were produced by the intersection of the laser beam with the edge of a cuvette which caused a brilliant flash of light. Other field designs were tested in an attempt to correct this problem. These fields prevented the light flash from reaching the detector, but resulted in a decrease in the signal-to-noise ratio. A rectangular dark field, centered on the disc as shown in Figure 3B, provided an acceptable signal-to-noise ratio and eliminated the asymmetrical signal.

The stability of a laser-modified centrifugal analyzer was tested by measuring the light scattered from a stable starch suspension at 30-s intervals over a 5-minute time period. The mean relative standard deviation (RSD) for a 5-minute interval for 14 cuvettes was 0.68%, which demonstrates exceptional instrument stability.

The earliest approach to automated nephelometric techniques was the use of continuous flow systems (Technicon Instruments, Co., Tarrytown, N.Y. 10591). Continuous flow techniques provide excellent timing of standards and samples, and it is a simple matter to keep the equipment free of contaminating reagents. Complex multichannel systems have been used in the author's laboratory and are capable of measurement of several antigens simultaneously. A simple system is shown in Figure 4 (Britain et al, 1977), a multi-use manifold for serum, urine, and cerebrospinal fluid analysis. The system consists of a sampler, proportionating pump, time delay coils, fluoronephelometer with 355nm filters, flow-through cuvette, and recorder. This system is not adaptable to rate measurements, but gives excellent results with equilibrium analyses. Some continuous flow systems use a predilution circuit; however, the author has found it more convenient to make any predilution of the sample with a semi-automated dilutor.

5. Procedures

The early manual methods using nephelometric techniques involved con-

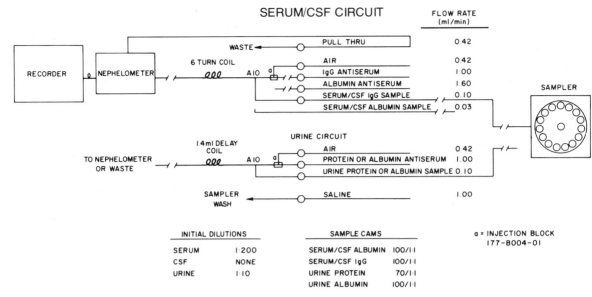

Fig. 4

Multi-use continuous flow manifold for measurement of specific proteins in serum, CSF, and urine.

(Reprinted by permission from Advances in Automated Analysis, Mediad Inc., pp. 274-277, (1977).

ventional fluorometers for the final detection of the complexes and used equilibrium measurements without polymer enhancement. Methods were developed for the measurement of specific proteins in serum, urine, and cerebrospinal fluid that involved an initial dilution of the sample followed by gentle mixing with diluted antiserum and incubation for 15-60 minutes to allow the Ag/Ab reaction to attain equilibrium. Serum blanks without antiserum were required and light-scattering measurements were made in a fluorometer. Light-scattering readings of blanks were subtracted from those of reactions containing Ag/Ab complexes. A multipoint standard curve was constructed and concentrations of unknown samples were obtained by interpolation from this standard curve.

The earlier manual methods did not contain PEG in the reaction medium, and a relatively long period of time was required for the reaction to achieve equilibrium. Similar approaches have been implemented recently using nephelometers with laser excitation sources with times of one to three hours being required for incubation in the absence of PEG. In the presence of PEG, these times are cut down to 30 minutes (Buffone et al, 1977).

The first kinetic procedures which were developed employed centrifugal analyzers. As described earlier, Tiffany et al (1974) used a fixed-time kinetic approach with readings at 6 and 60 seconds on a miniaturized centrifugal analyzer adapted for 90° light-scattering measurements. Methods for serum IgG, IgM, C3, and α_1-antitrypsin were described. The rate of the reaction was controlled by varying the amount of PEG in solution. A concentration of PEG of 20 g/liter was used to enable the reaction to proceed to equilibrium quickly enough for convenient analysis time, but still allowing for the use of an early reading.

Fixed-time kinetics can provide for increased throughput and improved precision. In a pseudo-first-order reaction, the change in absorbance between two fixed times is directly proportional to concentration. In monitoring the aggregation phase of an antigen-antibody reaction by light-scattering measurements, the change in intensity (ΔI) is not directly proportional to antigen concentration. However, a plot of ΔI versus antigen concentration displays characteristics of the precipitin curve and can be used as an analytical working curve. Advantages of such a kinetic approach are the speed of analysis, which is often less than two minutes, and the elimination of separate sample blank measurements.

Similar procedures have been developed in the author's laboratory for the laser-modified centrifugal analyzer (Buffone *et al*, 1975; White *et al*, 1976) with determinations of IgG, IgA, IgM, and C3 and C4 being made using a fixed-time kinetic approach as follows:

IgG: Samples and standards were initially diluted (100 fold) with phosphate-buffered saline (PBS) containing 4% PEG. A $250\mu l$ volume of diluted anti-human IgG was transferred to the reagent wells of the transfer disc, and $50\mu l$ of the diluted samples and standards and an additional $200\mu l$ of PEG-PBS diluent were transferred to the sample wells. After initiation of the reaction and initial mixing of reactants, the solutions were again mixed for 0.5 s, 5 s before each reading. Using the fixed-time kinetic approach, the light-scatter readings were taken 100 s apart ($t_1 = 15$ s, $t_2 = 115$ s).

IgA: The procedure for the measurement of IgA differed from that described for IgG only in the initial sample dilution (40 fold).

IgM: Initial sample dilution (15 fold) was in physiological saline. Reagent (diluted antiserum), diluent, and sample volumes were the same as those used to measure IgG. The fixed-time interval chosen for analysis was 170 s ($t_1 = 15$ s, $t_2 = 185$ s).

C3: Initial sample dilution (20 fold) was in physiologic saline; otherwise, the conditions were the same as for IgG. The fixed-time interval chosen for analysis was 140 s ($t_1 = 10$ s, $t_2 = 150$ s).

C4: Initial sample dilution (nine fold) was in physiologic saline and the fixed-time interval was 300 s with pooled human serum assayed ($t_1 = 10$ s, $t_2 = 310$ s).

Standardization for all protein assays was accomplished by use of commercial reference sera.

Standard curves of change in relative intensity (ΔI) between t_1 and t_2 to concentration of antigen again followed a similar pattern to conventional precipitin curves. The Beckman rate nephelometer uses a similar approach and monitors continuously the rate of formation of the complexes with approximately two minutes being required for each analysis.

Continuous flow systems have been used more extensively than any other light-scattering technique for specific protein measurement. Initial procedures were carried out in 0.9% saline or phosphate-buffered saline, but the use of PEG now has become widespread and offers advantages of speed of analysis and sensitivity over the use of saline alone. In the continuous flow methods, the Ag/Ab reaction is allowed to achieve equilibrium before the light-scattering measurement is made. Blanks must also be run to correct for intrinsic light-scattering of the biological samples. Non-linear standard curves are constructed in a manner similar to the manual methods. The rate of analysis usually is 60 samples per hour, but the necessity of blank measurements halves the throughput.

6. Detection of Antigen Excess Samples

All of the analytical methods have the inherent problem of requiring the detection of antigen excess samples. The precipitin curve shown in Figure 1 demonstrates that two widely varying antigen concentrations will give the same light-scattering response. One concentration is in antibody excess and the other in antigen excess. Since the standard curve is constructed in the zone of antibody excess, it is imperative that antigen excess samples be detected in order that dilution of the sample can be made. The manual discrete sample and centrifugal fast analyser methods can only detect antigen excess through a dilution of all samples to see if the response characterizes an antibody or an antigen excess zone. In practice, for serum proteins, the method conditions can be adjusted so that zone electrophoresis can be used to screen for those samples which might exhibit antigen excess for any specific protein. In many laboratories, serum samples for protein measurements are subjected to agarose gel electrophoresis, and only in the case of patients with profound hyperimmunoglobulinemia, such as in plasma cell dyscrasias, will antigen excess occur. For urine and CSF proteins it is advisable to screen for antigen excess using the dilution method.

Continuous flow analysis possesses a convenient means of detecting antigen excess since these samples will give a bimodal recorder peck. This bimodal response is caused by a gradient dilution of sample as it enters the antiserum stream. Thus, the reaction starts in antibody excess but soon achieves antigen excess.

7. Standardization

No primary standards exist for nephelometric assays; this is a common difficulty of all methods for measuring specific proteins. Where possible, secondary standards in a serum matrix which have been standardized against the International Reference Standard prepared by the World Health Organization should be used.

8. Sensitivity Limits of Nephelometry

Many variables enter into estimation of sensitivity limits of nephelometry such as the nature of the antigen, clarity of the specimen, etc. Using the laser nephelometer, limits of detection of IgE and C-reactive protein in serum approach 10^{-10} M (Russeau).

9. Applications of Nephelometry

A wide variety of analyses have been adapted to the nephelometric technique. A listing of applications from one commercial source (Hyland Diagnostics, Division of Travenol Laboratories, Costa Mesa, Calif. 92626) is shown in Table I.

Table I

METHODS DEVELOPED FOR LASER NEPHELOMETER

IMMUNOGLOBULINS	COMPLEMENT	ACUTE PHASE PROTEIN
IgG	C3	C-Reactive Protein
IgA	C4	α_1-Acid Glycoprotein
IgM	C3PA	α_1-Antitrypsin
IgD	C1q	Ceruloplasmin

COAGULATION	AUTO-IMMUNE	CARRIER PROTEINS
Plasminogen	Rheumatoid Factor	Ceruloplasmin
Antithrombin III		Haptoglobin
		Transferrin
		Prealbumin
		Albumin
		TBG

PROTEASE INHIBITORS	CSF	MISCELLANEOUS
α_1-Antitrypsin	IgG	CSF Total Protein
α_2-Macroglobulin	Albumin	Urine Total Protein
C1 Esterase Inhibitor		Amylase
		Lipase
		Triglycerides
		Antiserum Titer
		Human Plasma Fibrinogen

It is evident from this extensive list that this technically simple analytical system has immense potential.

10. Conclusion

Many factors must be taken into consideration in choosing a system for the nephelometric measurement of specific proteins. Since the standard curve is non-linear, several standards are required, and the tedium of analyzing all of the standards as well as unknowns makes automated techniques appear extremely attractive. The choice between continuous flow and kinetic discrete sample analytical techniques will depend upon the availability of equipment. Both have advantages and disadvantages. The continuous flow methods require sample blanks but offset this inconvenience by providing ready detection of antigen excess samples. The kinetic centrifugal fast analyzer procedures do not require blanks but require a separate analysis for detecting antigen excess. Some innovative development obviously is necessary to detect antigen excess for these kinetic techniques, and it is possible that monitoring reaction rates over the first few seconds of the reaction might be used. It has been demonstrated (Savory et al, 1974) that reactions carried out with antigen in large excess exhibit a very rapid initial rate (0-5 s) which subsequently becomes constant, while a reaction in which the antigen concentration is low (antibody excess) proceeds much slower initially (0-5 s), but continues to show increases in light-scattering over a longer time period.

Polymer enhancement of reactions increases both the speed and sensitivity of the Ag/Ab reaction and now is used with all systems. The angle of measurement usually is 90° although advantages of increased sensitivity come with other angles; one centrifugal fast analyzer system employs 180° as the angle of measurement.

Because of the sensitivity, simplicity, and low consumption of antiserum, the use of nephelometric methods for measuring specific proteins should continue to increase in popularity. The precision of the technique is excellent and greatly enhances the clinical value of specific protein measurements in biological fluids.

11. References

Alper, C. A. (1971). *In* "Advan. Automat., Anal., Technicon International Congress 1970" (Barton, E. C. *et al*, eds.) p. 13, Thurman Assoc., Miami

Alper, C. A., Propp, R. P., Klemperer, M. R. and Rosen, F. S. (1969). *J Clin Invest* **48**, 553

Boyden, A., Bolton, E. and Gemeroy, D. (1947). *J Immunol* **57**, 211

Britain, C. E., Butts, J. D. and Killingsworth, L. M. (1977). *In* "Advances in Automated Analysis" (Barton, E. C. *et al*, eds.) pp. 274-77, Mediad, Tarrytown, New York

Buffone, G. J., Cross, R. E., Savory, J. and Soodak, C. (1974). *Anal Chem* **46**, 2047

Buffone, G. J., Heintges, M. G., Savory, J. and Killingsworth, L. M. (1975). *Clin Chem* **21**, 943

Buffone, G. J., Lewis, S., Savory, J. and Hicks, J. M. (1977). *In* "Seminar on Proteins and Proteinopathies" (Sunderman, F. W., Sr., ed.) pp. 73-79, Institute for Clinical Science

Buffone, G. J., Savory, J. and Cross, R. E. (1974). *Clin Chem* **20**, 1320

Buffone, G. J., Savory, J., Cross, A. E. and Hammond, J. E. (1975). *Clin Chem* **21**, 1731

Buffone, G. J., Savory, J. and Hermans, J. (1975). *Clin Chem* **21**, 1735

Clarke, M. H. G. and Freeman, T. (1968). *Clin Sci* **35**, 403

Eckman, I., Robbins, J. B., Van den Hamer, C. J. A., Lentz, J. and Scheinberg, I. H. (1970). *Clin Chem* **16**, 558

Fahey, J. L. and McKelvey, E. M. (1965). *J Immunol* **94**, 84

Goettsch, E. and Kendall F. E. (1935). *J Biol Chem* **109**, 221

Goettsch, K. and Reeves, E. B. (1936). *J Clin Invest* **15**, 173

Grabar, P. and Burtin, P. (1964). "Immuno-electrophoretic analysis; applications to human biological fluids," Elsevier, New York

Grabar, P. and Williams, C. A. (1953). *Biochem Biophys Acta* **10**, 193

Heidelberger, M. and Kendall, F. E. (1929). *J Exp Med* **50**, 809

Heidelberger, M. and Kendall, F. E. (1932). *J Exp Med* **55**, 555

Heidelberger, M., Kendall, F. E. and Teorell, T. (1936). *J Exp Med* **63**, 819

Hellsing, K. (1972). *Colloquium on A.I.P. and Technicon International Congress* 17

Kabat, E. A., Glusman, M. and Knaub, V. (1948). *Amer J Med* **4**, 653

Kendall, F. E. (1938). *Cold Spring Harbor Symposia on Quantitative Biology* **6**, 376

Killingsworth, L. M. and Savory, J. (1971). *Clin Chem* **17**, 936

Killingsworth, L. M. and Savory, J. (1972). *Clin Chem* **18**, 335

Killingsworth, L. M. and Savory, J. (1973a). *Clin Chem* **19**, 403

Killingsworth, L. M. and Savory, J. (1973b). *Clin Chem Acta* **43**, 279

Killingsworth, L. M., Savory, J. and Teague, P. O. (1971). *Clin Chem* **17**, 374

Larson, C., Orenstein, P. and Ritchie, R. F. (1971). *In* "Advan. Automat. Anal. Technicon International Congress 1970" (Barton, E. C. *et al*, eds.) p. 9, Thurman Assoc., Miami

Laurell, C. B. (1965). *Anal Biochem* **10**, 358

Laurell, C. B. (1966). *Anal Biochem* **15**, 45

Leone, C. A. (1971). *In* "Methods in Immunology and Immunochemistry, III" (Williams, C. A. and Chase, M. W., eds.) pp. 86-94, Academic Press, New York

Li, I. W. and Williams, C. A. (1971). *In* "Methods in Immunology and Immuno-chemistry, III" (Williams, C. A. and Chase, M. W., eds.) pp. 94-102, Academic Press, New York

Lou, K. and Shanbron, E. (1967). *J Amer Med Assoc* **200**, 323

Mancini, G., Carbonara, A. O. and Heremans, J. F. (1965). *Immunochemistry* **2**, 235

Oudin, J. (1946). *C R Acad Sci* **222**, 115

Ritchie, R. F. (1967). *J Lab Clin Med* **70**, 512

Ritchie, R. F. and Graves, J. (1971). *In* "Advan. Automat., Anal. Technicon International Congress 1970" (Barton, E. C. *et al*, eds.) p. 25, Thurman Assoc., Miami

Russeau, R. J. Personal communication

Savory, J. and Killingsworth, L. M. (1973). *Annals of Clin Lab Sci* **3**, 43

Savory, J., Buffone, G. J. and Reich, R. (1974). *Clin Chem* **20**, 1071

Savory, J., Heintges, M. G., Killingsworth, L. M. and Potter, J. M. (1972). *Clin Chem* **18**, 37

Scheidegger, J. J. (1955). *Intern Arch Allergy Appl Immunol* **7**, 103

Schultze, H. E. and Schwick, G. (1959). *Clin Chem Acta* **4**, 15

Tiffany, T. O., Parella, J. M., Johnson, W. F. and Burtis, C. A. (1974). *Clin Chem* **20**, 1055

Wegfahrt, P. F., Fish, M. B., Aldana, F. B. and Aronson, S. B. (1971). *In* "Advan. Automat. Anal. Technicon International Congress 1970" (Barton, E. C. *et al*, eds.) p. 21, Thurman Assoc., Miami

White, R. E., Buffone, G. J., Savory, J. and Killingsworth, L. M. (1976). *Annals of Clin Lab Sci* **6**, 525

Acknowledgments

The author wishes to acknowledge the contributions of his colleagues Drs. G. M. Buffone and L. M. Killingsworth, whose work plays a prominent role in this present review.

CHAPTER **III**

Future Trends and Applications of Immunoprecipitin Techniques

R. F. RITCHIE, M.D.

Table of Contents

1. Introduction

The process by which immunoprecipitation occurs has been recognized since the late 1880's, but its advance out of the nineteenth century for practical purposes was delayed until 50 years after the chronological event. Evolution of protein analysis from the original manual, in-gel techniques to automation and sophisticated electronics has taken seven years. It should have taken only three. The recent burst of interest has resulted from the availability of several instruments of varying sophistication and of reagents specifically tailored for the applications (Tables I, II). The latter, the availability of appropriate reagents, has not always been the case. Until recently, manufacture of antisera was reminiscent of the "cottage industries," with most workers making their own materials. Commercial efforts were minimal at best, and advances came primarily from the academic sector. The noncompetitive approach of antiserum suppliers was based largely on the fact that the user was, in general, unsophisticated. Virtually anyone with two goats and a letterhead went into business, producing what was alleged to be usable antiserum.

Several events occurred during the early 1970's which resulted in a change, hopefully for the better. The introduction of the Automated Immunoprecipitin System made it possible to evaluate the performance of an antiserum in a strictly mechanical and unbiased fashion. The comparison of reagents, therefore, became a meaningful exercise, and in 1972, a group from the Center for Disease Control in Atlanta, Georgia, led by Dr. Charles Reimer, published an evaluation of commercial antisera which further documented the fact that buying antiserum was, at best, a "pig in a poke" situation in spite of the manufacturer's claim. Some reagents were totally devoid of activity, while others were only bordering on the satisfactory. None could match reagents that were made by knowledgeable laboratory personnel with an interest in the subject. It is perhaps these poor commercial reagents that were the major deterrents to developing satisfactory immunoprecipitin assays.

Since nephelometric analysis was the mode on which the original immunoprecipitin system was based, it has received a considerable amount of attention. It has been reviewed extensively, and, rather than attempt to condense the many articles or to author yet another manuscript summarizing the subject, an organized compendium of recent publications on the subject is given below to assist the interested reader.

2. Annotated References

A. General

Ritchie, R. F.: Automated immunoprecipitin analysis of serum proteins. *In* Putnam, F. W. (ed.): *The Plasma Proteins*. Vol. 2, 2nd edition, Academic Press, New York, pp. 375-425, 1975.

The chapter contains a historical review of events leading up to continuous flow nephelometry. The principles and mechanics of in-liquid continuous flow immunoanalysis are discussed. Examples of the mathematics of data reduction are given.

13 illustrations, 3 tables, 114 references.

Ritchie, R. F. (ed): *Automated Immunoanalysis*. Vol. 1 & 2, Dekker, New York, 1978.

The two-volume set extensively describes the theory and practice of nephelometric immunoassay.

19 chapters, 469 pages devoted to nephelometry alone.

Table I

DEDICATED INSTRUMENTS FOR SPECIFIC PROTEIN ANALYSIS

Company	Test/ Hour	Time	Name	Instrument Cost (1979)		Cost/ Test (1979)	Comment
a. Technicon Instrument Corporation	120	3 min	AIP		$14,000-$20,000 (two channel)	-$0.75-$1.00	Continuous Flow, End-Point Nephelometry
b. Hyland	60-70	1-2 h	PDQ	Neph. DP Diluter Transport System	$7,200 $4,500 $1,500 $4,500 $17,150	$0.67-$1.20	Manual, End-Point Nephelometry
c. International Diagnostic Technology	60	1 h	FIAX	Fluoro DP Diluter System	$7,250 $4,950 $1,650 $12,700	$1.50-$1.74	Manual, Fluorescence and solid phase
d. Behring Diagnostics	30-35	1-2 h	BD Laser		$12,000**-$100,000	$0.50-$1.50	Manual, End-Point Nephelometry
e. Beckman Instruments Inc.	30-40	20-80 s	ICS	System	$12,500++	$.80	Manual Rate Nephelometry
f. Kallestad Laboratories	30-40	1 h	LSA	Neph. System	$3,000 $10,000	$1.00	Manual, low cost device, nephelometer
g. Oxford Labs+	22	2 min	LINA		$22,000	$0.95	Kinetic or end-point nephelometry

*Instrument configuration variable—partial breakdown given
**Discount on basic system to $7,600
+Availability uncertain—possibly late 1979
++Multiple sample transport and data processor available early 1980

Table II

35 DISTRIBUTORS OF PLASMA PROTEIN ANTISERA

1. Alpha Gamma Labs	
2. Antibodies Incorporated	
3. Atlantic Antibodies	Principle
	Manufacturer
4. BBL	
5. Beckman Instruments	*Instrument
6. Behring Diagnostics	*Instrument/
	Major Supplier/
	Manufacturer
7. Bio-Rad	
8. Bioware	
9. Boehringer Manneheim	
10. Cal Biochem	
11. Cappel Laboratories	
12. Cordis	
13. Dade	
14. DaKopatts	
15. Gateway Immunosera	
16. Helena Laboratories	
17. Hyland	*Instrument/
	Major Supplier/
	Manufacturer
18. ICN Medical Diagnostics	
19. Janus Labs	
20. Kallestad	
21. Kent Laboratories	
22. Laboratory Diagnostics	
23. Lee Labs	
24. Litton-Bionetics	
25. Meloy	Major Supplier/
	Manufacturer
26. Miles	Major Supplier/
	Manufacturer
27. Millipore	
28. Nordic	
29. Orion	
30. Oxford	
31. Schwarz/Mann	
32. Spectrum Medical	
Instruments	
33. Tago Inc.	
34. Technicon Instrument	*Instrument
Corp.	
35. Wellcome	

B. Optics

Kusnetz, J. and Mansberg, H. P.: Optical considerations: Nephelometry. *In* Ritchie, R. F. (ed.): *Automated Immunoanalysis.* Vol. 1, Dekker, New York, pp. 1-43, 1978.

This large chapter includes an extensive and complete review of the optics involved in light-scattering analysis. It is well illustrated and is written in very readable fashion. It is a must for workers in the field.

19 illustrations, 1 table, 20 references.

C. Enhancing Agents

Hellsing, K.: Enhancing affects of nonionic polymers on immunochemical reactions. *In* Ritchie, R. F. (ed.): *Automated Immunoanalysis.* Vol. 1, Dekker, New York, pp. 67-112, 1978.

This 45-page chapter represents the most complete discussion and review of materials known to enhance immunologic reactions. It leaves no stone unturned.

164 references.

D. System Variables

Keren, D. F., Frye, R. M., Datiles, T. B., and Grindon, A. J.: A modification of the automated immunoprecipitin method for quantitation of human serum immunoglobulins. *Am J Clin Path*, **70**:41-44, 1978.

4 illustrations, 11 references.

Killingsworth, L. M.: Analytical variables for specific protein analysis. *In* Ritchie, R. F. (ed.): *Automated Immunoanalysis.* Vol. 1, Dekker, New York, pp. 113-137, 1978.

This paper discusses the technical and chemical parameters that affect protein immunoanalysis and are under the control of the laboratorian.

14 illustrations, 3 tables, 24 references.

E. Fast Analyzers

Savory, J. and Buffone, G. J.: The measurement of specific proteins by fast analysis techniques. *In* Ritchie, R. F.

(ed.): *Automated Immunoanalysis.* Vol. 2, Dekker, New York, pp. 335-352, 1978.

The authors describe the evolution of kinetic nephelometric analysis and the differences between rate and endpoint forms of analysis.

11 illustrations, 2 tables, 20 references.

F. Rate Nephelometry

Anderson, R. J. and Sternberg, J. C.: A rate nephelometer for immunoprecipitin measurement of specific serum proteins. *In* Ritchie, R. F. (ed.): *Automated Immunoanalysis.* Vol. 2, Dekker, New York, pp. 409-469, 1978.

Included in this chapter is an extensive discussion of rate nephelometry and of microprocessor controlled manual rate analysis of specific proteins.

26 illustrations, 2 tables.

Nishi, H. H. and Young, D. S.: A flexible reaction rate analytical system for the rapid determination of IgA, IgG, and IgM concentrations. *In* Ritchie, R. F. (ed.): *Automated Immunoanalysis.* Vol. 2, Dekker, New York, pp. 353-373, 1978.

The authors discuss the measurement of immunoglobulins by analyzing the rate of antigen-antibody complex formation. Special equipment is described.

14 illustrations, 6 references.

Sternberg, J. C.: The rate nephelometer for measuring specific proteins in immunoprecipitin reactions. *Clin Chem,* **23**:1456-1464, 1977.

This article gives an excellent review of rate nephelometry. Although the subject matter is general, it also focuses on a new commercially available Beckman instrument.

9 illustrations, 4 tables, 16 references.

G. Manual Instruments

Daigneault, R. and Lemieux, D.: Evaluation of a Behring laser-nephelometer

prototype in the measurement of IgG, IgA and IgM. *Clin Biochem,* **11**:28-31, 1978.

This paper describes some of the practical aspects of immunoglobulin analysis with a commercially available laser-nephelometer. Correlations between RID and nephelometry values are given.

6 illustrations, 3 tables, 1 reference.

Deaton, C. D., Maxwell, K. W., Smith, R. S., and Creveling, R. L.: Use of laser nephelometry in the measurement of serum proteins. *Clin Chem,* **22**:1465-1471, 1976.

The article describes in detail the workings of a commercially available nephelometer.

9 illustrations.

Deaton, C. D., Maxwell, K. W., and Smith, R. S.: Laser nephelometry. *In* Ritchie, R. F. (ed.): *Automated Immunoanalysis.* Vol. 2, Dekker, New York, pp. 375-407, 1978.

This paper gives a complete description of the application of laser light sources to nephelometry in the manual mode, with particular attention to the Hyland instrument.

18 illustrations, 6 tables, 21 references.

Sieber, A. and Gross, J.: Protein determination by laser nephelometry. *Medical Laboratory,* **2**:17-24, 1977.

The authors describe the use of the Behring laser nephelometer for the analysis of 6 major serum proteins. Precision data is included.

4 illustrations, 4 tables, 5 references.

Virella, G. and Fudenberg, N. H.: Comparison of immunoglobulin determination in pathological sera by radial immunodiffusion and laser nephelometry. *Clin Chem,* **23**:1925-1928, 1977.

A study of a small number of patients confirms that optical methods are less affected by physical parameters than are those performed by gel-diffusion.

2 tables, 19 references.

Ellis, D. and Buffone, G. J.: New approach to evaluation of proteinuric states. *Clin Chem*, **23**:666-670, 1977.

A potentially extremely important upgrading of urinalysis by specific protein measurement is described employing nephelometry.

1 illustration, 6 tables, 9 references.

H. Nephelometric Inhibition

Cambiaso, C. L., Masson, P. L., Vaerman, J. P., and Heremans, J. F.: Automated nephelometric immunoassay (ANIA). I. Importance of antibody affinity. *J Immunol Methods*, **5**:153-163, 1974.

The workers describe their efforts at fractionating antibody according to affinity, making use of solid phase immunoadsorbant technology.

9 illustrations, 21 references.

Cambiaso, C. L., Riccomi, H., Masson, P. L., and Heremans, J. F.: Automated nephelometric immunoassay. II. Its application to the determination of hapten. *J Immunol Methods*, **5**:293-302, 1974.

This publication describes refinements of the nephelometric inhibition assay which the authors developed in 1971. Their techniques are applied to several haptens.

8 illustrations, 10 references.

Gauldie, J. and Bienenstock, J.: Automated nephelometric analysis of haptens. *In* Ritchie, R. F. (ed.): *Automated Immunoanalysis*. Vol. 1., Dekker, New York, pp. 321-333, 1978.

This review paper addresses the subject of nephelometric inhibition immunoassay as it has been employed by the authors to measure a wide range of haptens, including digoxin and morphine.

3 illustrations, 41 references.

Ritchie, R. F. and Stevens, J.: A nephelometric inhibition modification for rate analysis of specific proteins. *Protides Biol Fluids*, **25**:433-436, 1977.

The paper describes the application of inhibition nephelometry to rate analysis of IgE, illustrating the substantial increase in sensitivity.

3 illustrations, 5 references.

I. New Applications

Borgen, J., and Ramslo, I.: Lysozyme determination in serum or urine by a simple nephelometric method. *Clin Chem*, **23**:1599-1601, 1977.

An interesting application of light-scattering analysis to both enzymology and bacteriology.

4 illustrations, 12 references.

Goodswaard, J. and Virella, G.: Immunochemical determination of human lysozyme by laser nephelometry. *Clin Chem*, **23**:967-970, 1977.

An extension of the paper cited above. The article employs specific antiserum for the nephelometric assay, and correlation with the lytic assay is given.

2 illustrations, 2 tables, 12 references.

Grange, J., Roch, A. M., and Quash, G. A.: Nephelometric assay of antigens and antibodies with latex particles. *J Immunol Methods*, **18**:365-375, 1977.

These workers describe immobilization of antigen or antibody to particles and the modulating effect of changing various parameters on the antigen-antibody reactions as examined in a fluorometer employed as a nephelometer. Excellent sensitivity was achieved with several systems.

9 illustrations, 6 references.

Hamers, N. N., Donker-Koopman, W. E., Reijngoad, D.-J., Schram, A. W., and Tager, J. M.: An optical method for the detection of antibodies to glycosphingolipids and other antigens. *Immunochemistry*, **15**:97-105, 1978.

5 illustrations, 2 tables, 29 references.

J. Special Applications

Automated Immunoanalysis, Part I., Ritchie, R. F. (ed.): Dekker, New York, 1978.

Albumin, Smith, L., 181-201.
5 illustrations, 10 tables, 40 references.

Complement (C3), Pinsker, M.C., 285-293.
4 illustrations, 5 tables, 15 references.

IgA, Dionne, J. A. and Peoples, C. A., 227-237.
3 illustrations, 3 tables, 17 references.

IgM, Milford-Ward, A., 239-252.
7 illustrations, 4 tables, 14 references.

Immunoglobulins, Walker, W. H. C., and Gauldie, J., 203-225.
4 illustrations, 3 tables, 44 references.

Low-density Lipoproteins, Ritchie, R. F., 267-284.
8 illustrations, 25 references.

Transferrin, Daigneault, R., 253-266.
5 illustrations, 2 tables, 29 references.

Ballantyne, F. C., Williamson, J., Shapiro, D., Caslake, M. J., and Perry, B.: Estimation of apolipoprotein B in man by immunonephelometry. *Clin Chem*, **24**:788-792, 1978.

5 tables, 20 references.

Gilliland, B. C.: Immunologic quantitation of serum immunoglobulins. *Am J Clin Pathol*, **68**:664-670, 1977.

3 illustrations, 2 tables, 43 references.

CHAPTER **IV**

Standardization of Calibration Materials and Reagents for Specific Protein Analysis

L. M. KILLINGSWORTH, Ph.D.

Table of Contents

1. Introduction

Immunoprecipitin techniques have emerged as powerful analytical tools for the investigation of specific proteins in human serum, urine, and cerebrospinal fluid. Popular quantitative methods based on diffusion of antigen or antibody through a gel medium (Mancini et al, 1965; Fahey and McKelvey, 1965; Laurell, 1972) are now being supplemented by analytical approaches involving the measurement of light scattering from immunochemical reactions in aqueous medium (Killingsworth and Savory, 1971; Ritchie et al, 1973; Ritchie, 1975; Killingsworth, 1976). Growing clinical interest in protein data has led to widespread use of these techniques by many laboratories.

It has long been realized that interlaboratory comparability of specific protein results leaves much to be desired (Rowe et al, 1970). Results from a recent proficiency survey in Scandinavia emphasize the magnitude of the dilemma and point out some possible avenues for improvement (Landaas et al, 1978). In this study, a lyophilized human pool serum was assayed for 13 proteins by 98 laboratories. The proteins measured included immunoglobulins, complement components, transport proteins, protease inhibitors, and acute phase reactants. Survey samples were assayed as routine specimens with use of radial immunodiffusion, electroimmunoassay, automated nephelometry, and other, non-immunoprecipitin methods.

The best results were obtained for albumin, with an inter-laboratory coefficient of variation of 8.4%, even though this determination was carried out by the largest number of laboratories. This relatively small variation for albumin confirms results from a survey performed for the College of American Pathologists by Batsakis and coworkers in 1976 (Batsakis et al, 1976). They found inter-laboratory variability of from 7.3% to 10.0% for four samples assayed by over 1300 laboratories.

Results for the other twelve proteins in the Scandinavian study revealed inter-laboratory coefficients of variation ranging from 14.6% for Immunoglobulin G to 28.7% for haptoglobin. Other studies, limited to the major immunoglobulin classes, have reported similar large unacceptable variations between laboratories (Rowe et al, 1970; Rowe et al, 1973; CDC, 1973; Ferguson et al, 1974).

Since these differences are significantly greater than the analytical variability of the techniques employed, it would seem that parameters affecting accuracy should be considered. This paper will discuss standardization of calibration materials and reagents for immunoprecipitin methods as a means of maximizing accuracy and consistency of specific protein results.

2. Calibration Materials

A significant effort in the standardization of calibration materials has been carried out under the auspices of the World Health Organization (Rowe et al, 1970; Rowe et al, 1973). The WHO International Reference Preparations for Human Immunoglobulins IgG, IgA, and IgM has been distributed widely and employed with some success in decreasing inter-laboratory variability.

The arbitrary International Units for calibration of these preparations have not, however, been universally accepted (Reimer, 1972; Reimer and Maddison, 1976). Criticisms of this approach have centered around the lack of interpretive data based on International Units, though normal values have been published for pediatric as well as adult populations. Other criticisms are based on the belief that mass units are fundamentally acceptable and should not be abandoned.

In response to the demand for mass units, several investigators as well as reagent manufacturers have published factors for conversion of International Units into more conventional concentrations formats (Rowe *et al*, 1972; Reimer and Maddison, 1976; Buckley and Dorsey, 1971; Cejka *et al*, 1974; Pilgrim *et al*, 1975). When expressed as micrograms of immunoglobulin per 1.00 International Unit, these conversion factors range from 59.5 to 94.0 for IgG, from 10.0 to 43.1 for IgA, and from 3.06 to 8.70 for IgM. Clearly, unanimous agreement has not been reached. This could be due to differences in calibration standards and in reactivity of the antisera used by the various groups. Each conversion factor is, therefore, specific for the combination of materials used by each group and is of limited usefulness.

The WHO standard, due to its high turbidity, has not proved to be generally suitable for nephelometric techniques. To accommodate this analytical approach, as well as others, the immunoglobulin standard prepared by the International Federation of Clinical Chemistry has recently been calibrated against the WHO standard (Whicher *et al*, 1978). Results were reported for IgG, IgA, and IgM measured by electroimmunoassay and radial immunodiffusion, and IgG and IgA measured by nephelometry. The same antisera were used for all studies, which were performed by specialized laboratories. Under these conditions, inter-laboratory variability was small and units could be ascribed to the IFCC material for IgG, IgA, and IgM. The group involved in this study will now carry out further calibration of the IFCC standard with use of reference antiserum reagents. They also have published information on standard methodologies for calibration studies.

Even though work continues apace on immunoglobulin standardization, the remainder of the more than 100 plasma proteins have been somewhat neglected. Purified preparations of some proteins are routinely available, but doubts persist about possible changes in their antigenic character resulting from the purification process itself. In addition, experience has shown that analyses performed on biological fluids can better be standardized by use of calibration materials in a biological matrix. A serum-based material, calibrated for the major proteins of clinical interest and applicable for standardization of the commonly-employed immunoprecipitin methods, would constitute an important step toward reducing inter-laboratory variability.

3. Reagents

A. Assessment of Antibody Performance

Immunochemical quantitation of specific proteins requires strict monitoring of the biological reagents which are used. Preparations of animal immunoglobulins directed against human proteins must be characterized with respect to performance criteria in the analytical system of choice. Antibody performance characteristics which must be established and maintained include specificity, sensitivity, and reactivity in the region of antibody excess. It is also important to characterize the zones of antigen-antibody equivalence and antigen excess.

Specificity

Antiserum specificity can be defined as the difference in reactivity of the reagent for antigens of molecular structure similar to the analyte. Demonstration of differential reactivity for similar antigens is dependent upon the sensitivity of the methods chosen and is, therefore, a relative term. For this term to be meaningful, the method chosen to demonstrate specificity must have an equal or lower limit of detection for the antigen-antibody reaction than the analytical method. Currently, antiserum specificity is best assessed by use of gel diffusion

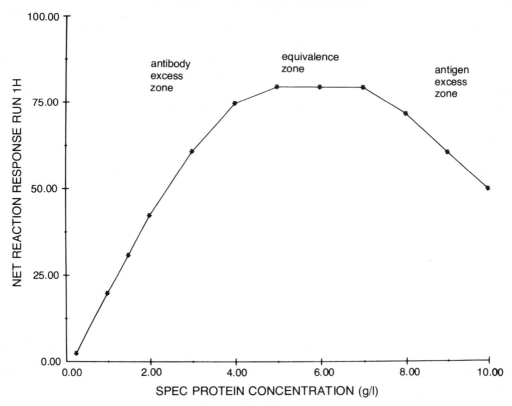

NEPHELOMETRIC PRECIPITIN CURVE

Fig. 1

NEPHELOMETRIC PRECIPITIN CURVE AT EQUILIBRIUM

(From: Killingsworth, L. M. and Killingsworth, C. E., Immunochemistry update: Profile of an evolving laboratory service. Laboratory Management, November, 1977, p. 36. Copyright 1977 by United Business Publications, Inc. and reproduced by permission of the copyright owner.)

techniques such as immunoelectrophoresis and Oucterlony double diffusion. The antiserum is allowed to react with a biological fluid known to contain the analyte as well as other protein components. The presence of a single precipitin reaction is evidence for monospecificity at the level of detection for these methods. This approach is by no means foolproof, but it does provide the analyst with a method for determining the suitability of a reagent to be used for quantitation of one protein in the presence of many others.

Sensitivity

The limit of detection, or sensitivity, of most gel diffusion methods can be described as the lowest concentration of antigen which gives a precipitate visible to the eye. Various other approaches, such as the use of radioisotopes and fluorescent labels, can be utilized to lower the detection limit. Sensitivity for photometric methods, such as immunonephelometry, is based on detection of a reaction peak above the background noise level. This lower limit of measurement is both reagent- and method-dependent, but can be a useful parameter to describe antibody reactivity at lower antigen concentrations when reaction conditions are kept constant.

The precipitin curve

Antibody reactivity over a wide range of antigen concentrations can be investigated through the precipitin curve (Killingsworth and Britain, 1977). The nephelometric precipitin curve, as shown in

Figure 1, will be presented as an example. The ordinate shows the blank-corrected light-scattering response at quasi-equilibrium with antigen concentration on the abscissa. This plot can be valuable in evaluating the general performance of an antiserum at a given dilution when reacting under a specified set of conditions. An indication of sensitivity can be obtained by noting response at low antigen levels. Characteristics of the analytical working curve, the antibody excess region, can also be determined. This can be important for deriving a curve-fitting algorithm for the method. The equivalence zone marks the upper limit of antigen concentration at which the antibody can be used for quantitation and is similar to antibody titer in some respects. Information concerning the region of antigen excess can be valuable in identifying samples containing elevated concentrations of antigen.

Effects of alterations in antigen-antibody ratio on the precipitin curve are shown in Figures 2 and 3 for trans-ferrin and haptoglobin model systems, respectively. In the transferrin studies, three antibody dilutions were allowed to react over a wide range of antigen concentration. Note the shift in the point of equivalence to higher antigen levels as well as absolute increases for light-scattering responses in the antibody excess zone as more antibody is made available for reaction. In the haptoglobin experiment, the antigen-antibody ratio was manipulated by changing the sample size while maintaining a constant antibody concentration. This resulted in a shift of equivalence to lower antigen concentrations with increased light-scattering response in the antibody excess zone as the amount of antigen in the reaction mixture increased. It is apparent from these investigations that any attempt to represent antibody performance in a nephelometric system in terms of "titer" must include antigen and antibody concentrations in the reaction mixture, in addition to data on light-scattering response and the location of the equivalence point.

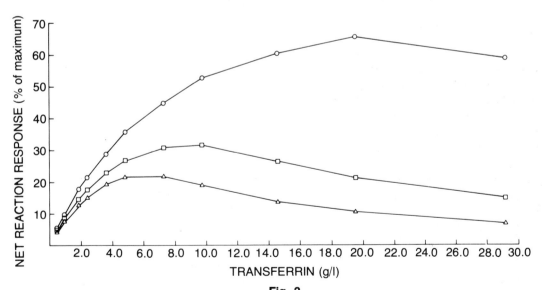

Fig. 2

EFFECTS OF ANTIBODY DILUTION ON THE PRECIPITIN CURVE

○ 50-fold antiserum dilution   □ 100-fold antiserum dilution   △150-fold antiserum dilution

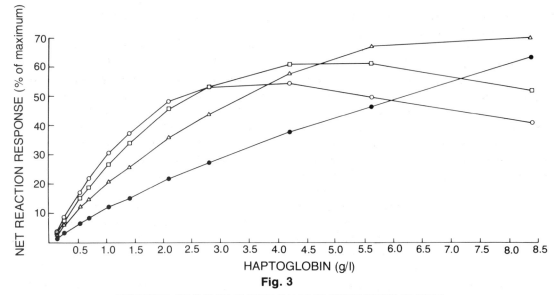

Fig. 3

EFFECTS OF SAMPLE SIZE ON THE PRECIPITIN CURVE

Relative sample size   1.00   0.70   0.43   0.22

                        ○   □   △   ●

(From: Killingsworth, L. M. and Killingsworth, C. E., Immunochemistry update: Profile of an evolving laboratory service. Laboratory Manage-ment, November, 1977, p. 36. Copyright 1977 by United Business Pub-lications, Inc. and reproduced by permission of the copyright owner.)

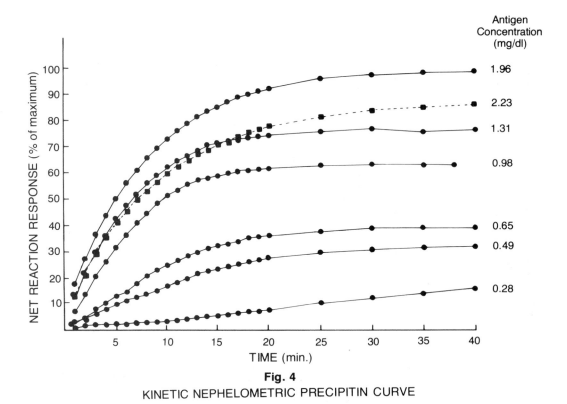

Fig. 4

KINETIC NEPHELOMETRIC PRECIPITIN CURVE

(From: Killingsworth, L. M. and Savory, J., Nephelometric studies of the precipitin reaction: A model system for specific protein measurements. Clin. Chem. 19, 403, 1973. Copyright 1973 by the American Association for Clinical Chemistry and reproduced by permission of the copyright owner.)

Figure 4 presents the precipitin curve from a kinetic standpoint and evaluates antibody performance with respect to time (Killingsworth and Savory, 1973). In this study, antigen concentrations ranging from distinct antibody excess to antigen excess were mixed with a constant amount of antibody. The initial reaction rates increased up to the point of equivalence and decreased in antigen excess. Thus, it can be seen that initial reaction rate, maximum reaction rate, or the time required to reach the maximum rate can be used for quantitative purposes (Killingsworth and Savory, 1973; Buffone *et al*, 1975; Sternberg, 1977). Proper reagent characterization for kinetic methods should include studies of reactions as a function of time for several antigen concentrations.

Long-term reagent monitoring

Reagent performance studies should not be limited to an initial antiserum evaluation. Long-term reagent quality control can help insure consistency of results by minimizing drift and detecting reagent instability. The first step in this process is to establish limits for acceptable reagent variability. Precipitin curve data for complement component C3, collected weekly over a period of six months, are shown in Figure 5. The points represent the mean reaction response for each standard while the brackets include plus and minus two standard deviations from the mean. With such limits of variability established, daily checks of the standard curve and weekly precipitin curve studies can help

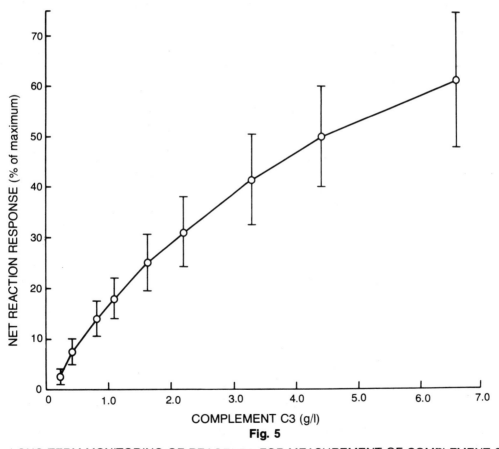

Fig. 5

LONG-TERM MONITORING OF REAGENTS FOR MEASUREMENT OF COMPLEMENT C3

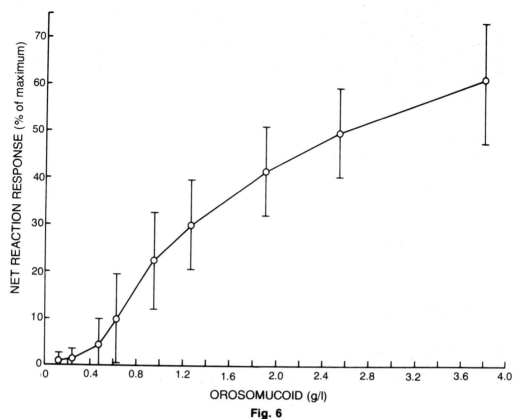

Fig. 6

LONG-TERM MONITORING OF REAGENTS FOR MEASUREMENT OF OROSOMUCOID

provide results which are comparable over a long period of time. Figure 6 depicts unacceptable performance in the antiserum reagent used to quantitate orosomucoid. Sensitivity is not sufficient with low normal levels, and the large standard deviations throughout the entire range are an indication of antiserum instability or inconsistency.

B. Reaction Conditions

Components other than the primary reactants must be considered as integral parts of immunoprecipitin analysis. Factors such as non-ionic polymers, neutral salts, and hydrogen ion concentration can have significant effects on complex formation, thereby influencing the precipitin curve and the final analytical result. Optimization of these factors should result in immunochemical techniques with improved sensitivity, accuracy, and precision, while standardization of op-

timized reaction conditions could be a significant step toward improving the over-all quality of results.

Effects of non-ionic polymers

A kinetic plot of a model antigen-antibody reaction is shown in Figure 7. Antigen and antibody were present in approximately equivalent proportions, and the reaction was carried out in three diluents: saline, a tris-chloride buffer of low ionic strength, and a saline solution containing polyethylene glycol (Mol. wt. 6,000) at a concentration of 40 g/l (Killingsworth et al, 1974). Results are plotted as a percent of the equilibrium light-scattering response. Reaction enhancement was achieved in either tris-chloride buffer or PEG, as compared with saline. It should be noted that the equilibrium light-scattering response was greatest with PEG, followed by tris-chloride and then saline.

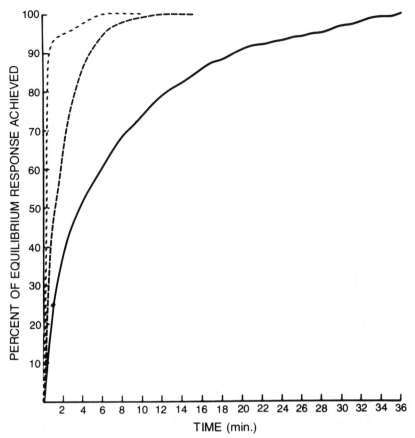

Fig. 7

KINETIC STUDIES OF THE IgG—ANTI-IgG REACTION WITH THREE DILUENTS

————— Saline   ————— Tris-Cl Buffer   ————— Polyethylene Glycol

(From: Killingsworth, L. M., Buffone, G. J., Sonawane, M. B., and Lunsford, G. C., Optimizing nephelometric measurement of specific serum proteins: Evaluation of three diluents. Clin. Chem. 20, 1548, 1974. Copyright 1974 by the American Association for Clinical Chemistry and reproduced by permission of the copyright owner.)

Lizana and Hellsing have shown effects of polymer on the nature of the precipitin curve (Lizana and Hellsing, 1974a; Lizana and Hellsing, 1974b; Hellsing, 1978). In their studies, using several proteins as model systems, significant enhancement of the equilibrium response was observed with PEG, but the apparent zone of equivalence was also shifted to higher antigen concentrations as the amount of PEG was increased. The enhancement effects and equivalence zone shift are probably due to changes in the size and/or number of the immune complexes in the presence of polymer (Hellsing, 1978).

Effects of salts

Neutral salts also have some effect on both the initial rate and the final net light-scattering response from immunoprecipitin reactions (Killingsworth and Savory, 1973; Killingsworth, 1978). Figure 8 shows a kinetic plot of a model antigen-antibody reaction carried out in 0.1 mol/liter solutions of sodium with four anions: fluoride, chloride, bromide, and nitrate. The initial reaction rate and equilibrium response were slightly enhanced with sodium fluoride as compared with chloride, bromide, and nitrate salts. Evaluation of these data is

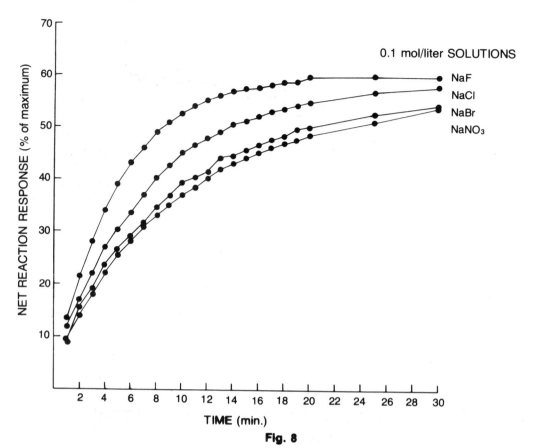

Fig. 8

EFFECTS OF 0.1 MOL/LITER SODIUM SALTS ON A MODEL ANTIGEN-ANTIBODY REACTION

aided by consideration of the hydration spheres of the anions studied. Relative enhancement takes place with those ions having larger hydration spheres. This could be the result of a "salting out" effect on the antigen-antibody complexes caused by ions binding available water. Thus, in the presence of an ion with a large hydration sphere, water is more easily excluded from the complexes as they form. Another possible mechanism postulates inhibition of the immunochemical reaction by ions with the same charge as the antigen. In this case, those anions which are least shielded by hydration spheres compete with the antigen for charged antibody binding sites.

Effects of pH

Studies on the effects of hydrogen ion concentration on a model IgG—anti-IgG system (Figure 9) showed only a slight enhancement of the equilibrium response at pH 6.72, as compared with solutions up to pH 7.67. The initial reaction rates were not significantly different. The pH factor must be considered, especially in the measurement of urinary proteins, since partial denaturation of the reactants at extremes of pH could result in inhibition of the immunochemical reaction, leading to inaccurate results.

C. Comparison of Commercial Reagents

Since most laboratories utilize antiserum reagents from commercial vendors, it is essential to assess reactivity of various products to determine their suitability for use with immunoprecipitin

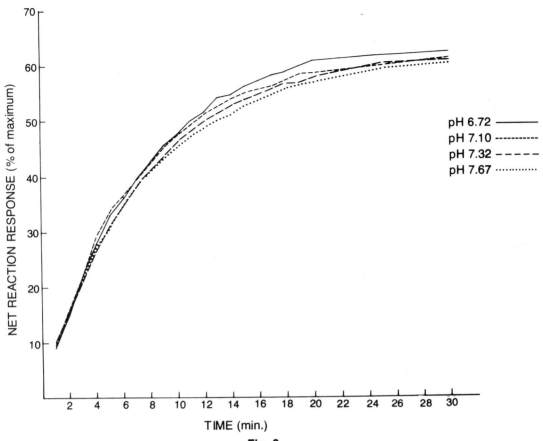

Fig. 9

INFLUENCE OF pH ON A MODEL ANTIGEN-ANTIBODY REACTION

methods. Reimer and colleagues evaluated the specificity of many commercial products for quantitation of immunoglobulins by radial immunodiffusion (Reimer, 1972; Reimer et al, 1970; Phillips et al, 1971). Even though their initial studies revealed lack of monospecificity for many reagents, follow-up studies showed marked improvement in quality of antisera.

Evaluation of antisera for nephelometric immunoprecipitin analysis by use of precipitin curves showed marked differences in some antisera, while others were comparable in performance (Killingsworth and Britain, 1977). Figure 10 shows precipitin curves for three commercial antisera to haptoglobin with antigen concentrations from 0.25 to 7.5 g/l. All three reagents were diluted 50-fold in PEG. Whereas the antiserum represented by the circles showed slightly higher reaction responses with low haptoglobin levels than the antiserum depicted with triangles, the latter reagent maintained antibody excess to higher levels. The antiserum shown with the squares reacted only slightly in the assay system. It should be emphasized that reactivity (or lack of it) in a nephelometric system does not necessarily result in similar reactivity in a gel medium. The vendor comparison for transferrin antiserum, shown in Figure 11, indicated clear superiority of the product represented by triangles, and

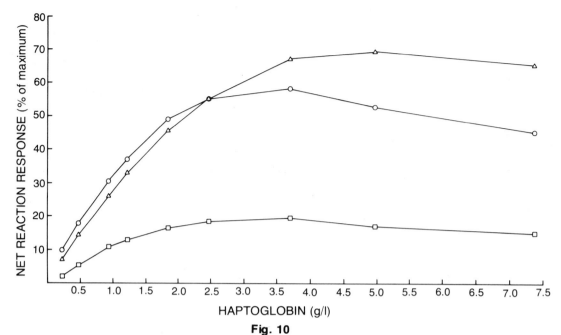

Fig. 10

COMPARISON OF THREE COMMERCIAL ANTISERUM REAGENTS FOR THE
DETERMINATION OF HAPTOGLOBIN

(From: Killingsworth, L. M. and Killingsworth, C. E., Immunochemistry update: Profile of an evolving laboratory service. Laboratory Management, November, 1977, p. 36. Copyright 1977 by United Business Publications, Inc. and reproduced by permission of the copyright owner.)

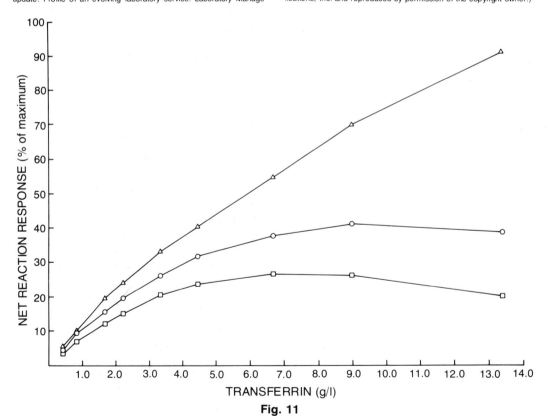

Fig. 11

COMPARISON OF THREE COMMERCIAL ANTISERUM REAGENTS FOR THE
DETERMINATION OF TRANSFERRIN

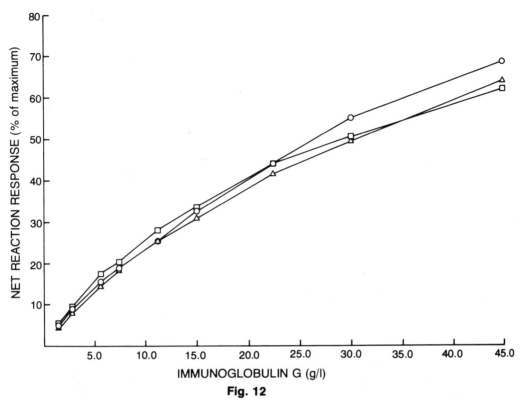

Fig. 12

COMPARISON OF THREE COMMERCIAL ANTISERUM REAGENTS FOR THE
DETERMINATION OF IgG

further suggested that a higher dilution of antiserum would be appropriate, since antigen excess was not even approached under the reaction conditions. Virtually no difference was seen in the three products for quantitation of IgG (Figure 12). This is surprising, since immunoglobulins exhibit such a remarkable degree of heterogeneity.

The current status of antiserum products by commercial vendors, as described by Reimer (Reimer, 1972; Reimer et al, 1970; Phillips et al, 1971) and as depicted in Figures 10-12, requires that each product be evaluated for specificity and reactivity by the analytical method in which they are to be used as reagents. Antisera available in kit form to be used with a specific instrument, as well as antisera marketed in bulk form for general use, should be clearly labeled as to these performance characteristics.

4. Summary and Conclusions

This paper has discussed factors affecting the accuracy of immunoprecipitin measurements of specific proteins and has attempted to recommend approaches for standardization of calibration materials and reagents.

1. Current international efforts for standardization of calibration materials are largely limited to the immunoglobulins. These efforts should be expanded to provide a generally useful serum-based material, calibrated for the higher concentration immunoglobulins, complement components, transport proteins, protease inhibitors, and acute phase reactants.

2. Laboratories should establish reagent performance standards for analytical specificity, sensitivity, reactivity, and long-term consistency. Both gel diffusion methods and nephelometric techniques can be utilized to establish criteria and monitor performance.

3. Immunoprecipitin analysis should be performed under standardized reaction conditions which are optimized for those factors which influence the formation of antigen-antibody complexes.

4. Commercial vendors should thoroughly document the performance of their antiserum products for each analytical method in which they are to be utilized. Results of reagent evaluations should be made readily available to consumers.

Attainment of accuracy for immunoprecipitin testing can only be achieved through the joint efforts of national or international health organizations, associations of laboratory professionals, reagent manufacturers, and individual clinical laboratories. Cooperation among all these groups is essential if significant advances are to be made in this area which promises to offer novel approaches for describing pathophysiological processes and aiding in the diagnosis of disease.

5. References

Batsakis, J. G., Aronsohn, R. S., Walker, W. A. and Barnes, B. (1976). *Am J Clin Pathol* **66**, 238

Buckley, C. E. and Dorsey, F. C. (1971). *Ann Intern Med* **75**, 679

Buffone, G. J., Savory, J., Cross, R. E. and Hammond, J. E. (1975). *Clin Chem* **21**, 1731

Cejka, J., Mood, D. W. and Kim, C. S. (1974). *Clin Chem* **20**, 656

Fahey, J. L. and McKelvey, E. M. (1965). *J Immunol* **94**, 84

Ferguson, A., Dick, H. M., Fallon, R. J., Logan, R. W. and Meudell, C. M. (1974). *Scot Med J* **19**, 113

Hellsing, D. (1978). *In* "Automated Immunoanalysis" (Ritchie, R. F., ed.) chap. 3, Marcel Dekker, New York

Killingsworth, L. M. (1976). *In* "Protides of the Biological Fluids," 23rd Colloquium 1975 (Peters, H., ed.) p. 291, Pergamon Press, New York

Killingsworth, L. M. (1978). *In* "Automated Immunoanalysis" (Ritchie, R. F., ed.) chap. 4, Marcel Dekker, New York

Killingsworth, L. M. and Britain, C. E. (1977). *Clin Chem* **23**, 1120

Killingsworth, L. M. and Savory, J. (1971). *Clin Chem* **17**, 936

Killingsworth, L. M. and Savory, J. (1973). *Clin Chem* **19**, 403

Killingsworth, L. M., Buffone, G. J., Sonawane, M. B. and Lunsford, G. C. (1974). *Clin Chem* **20**, 1548

Landaas, S., Skrede, S. and Eldjarn, L. (1978). *Scand J Clin Lab Invest* **38**, 295

Laurell, C. B. (1972). *Scand J Clin Lab Invest* **29**, *Suppl* **124**, 21

Lizana, J. and Hellsing, K. (1974a). *Clin Chem* **20**, 415

Lizana, J. and Hellsing, K. (1974b). *Clin Chem* **20**, 1181

Mancini, G., Carbonara, A. O. and Heremans, J. F. (1965). *Immunochemistry* **2**, 235

Phillips, D. J., Shore, S. L., Maddison, S. E., Gordon, D. S. and Reimer, C. B. (1971). *J Lab Clin Med* **77**, 639

Pilgrim, U., Fontanellaz, H. P., Evers, G. and Hitzig, W. H. (1975). *Helv Paediatr Acta* **30**, 121

"Proficiency testing: Non-syphilis serology. Quantitative immunoglobulins" (1973). Center for Disease Control, USPHS, U.S. Dept. of HEW, Atlanta

Reimer, C. B. (1972). *Health Lab Sci* **9**, 178

Reimer, C. B. and Maddison, S. E. (1976). *Clin Chem* **22**, 577

Reimer, C. B., Phillips, D. J., Maddison, S. E. and Shore, S. L. (1970). *J Lab Clin Med* **76**, 949

Ritchie, R. F. (1975). *In* "The Plasma Proteins," 2nd ed. (Putnam, F. W., ed.) chap. 8, Academic Press, New York

Ritchie, R. F., Alper, C. A. and Graves, J. (1973). *Am J Clin Pathol* **59**, 151

Rowe, D. S., Anderson, S. G. and Grab, B. A. (1970). *Bull WHO* **42**, 535

Rowe, D. S., Grab, B. and Anderson, S. G. (1972). *Bull WHO* **46**, 67

Sternberg, J. C. (1977). *Clin Chem* **23**, 1456

Whicher, J. T., Hunt, J., Perry, D. E., Hobbs, J. R., Fifield, R., Keyser, J., Riches, P., Smith, A. M., Thompson, R. A., Milford-Ward, A. and White, P. (1978). *Clin Chem* **24**, 531

PART 2

DIAGNOSTIC IMMUNOLOGY

CHAPTER **I**

Recent Developments in Homogeneous Immunoassay Techniques

R. S. SCHNEIDER, Ph.D., D. S. KABAKOFF, Ph.D.,
H. M. GREENWOOD, Ph.D.

Table of Contents

1. Introduction

Increasingly, immunoassay techniques are being used to quantitate many analytes of clinical interest including proteins, viruses, hormones, and exogenous drugs. The specific recognition of antigens by antibodies forms the basis for these methods. Various analytical systems which utilize different monitors of the reaction of immune components have been developed. This paper briefly reviews some recent developments in homogeneous immunoassays and then discusses one such method, the EMIT® homogeneous enzyme immunoassay, and its application to the measurement of drugs and haptens in body fluids in more detail.

Immunoassays may be classified according to the method used to detect the reaction between antibody (Ab) and antigen (Ag), described by the basic equation below:

$$Ag + Ab \rightarrow Ag \cdot Ab \qquad \textit{(Peetoom, 1971)}$$

The analyte of interest is most often the antigen; however, in principle, any of the components may be measured. Two basic classes of immunoassays exist:

Type I - those which employ no labeled reactant; and

Type II - those which employ a labeled reactant.

Assays of Type I have been used exclusively to measure proteins since precipitating complexes formed by proteins with their respective antibodies can be easily detected. The precipitation reaction is the basis of such well-established techniques as agglutination and immunodiffusion (Peetoom, 1971). More recently nephelometry, or light-scattering spectroscopy, has been used to quantitate proteins (Cohen and Benedek, 1975).

Either antigen, antibody, or both, may be labeled with an indicator molecule in Type II immunoassays. In reviewing recent developments in the field of homogeneous immunoassays, attention will be

confined to systems in which the antigen is labeled:

$$Ag + Ag\text{-}L + Ab \rightarrow Ag\text{-}L\cdot Ab + Ag\cdot Ab$$
$$L = Label$$

(Cohen and Benedek, 1975)

Competition between Ag (the sample) and labeled antigen (Ag-L) for a limited number of antibody binding sites results in a partitioning of the label between free and bound states. Measurement of either the free labeled antigen (Ag-L) or the antibody-bound label (Ag-L·Ab) allows quantitation of the antigen.

Before discussing the types of indicator molecules which have been employed, it is necessary to present one additional conceptual classification of immunoassays: the distinction between homogeneous and heterogeneous assays. This classification was introduced in 1972 by Rubenstein, Schneider and Ullman in their first paper on homogeneous enzyme immunoassay. As described above, quantitation of the analyte requires measurement of either the free or antibody-bound labeled antigen. If the properties of the free and bound labels are identical, a physical separation is required to distinguish them. An assay which requires separation is termed a heterogeneous assay. If the properties of the indicator molecule can be modulated by the antibody-antigen reaction, no separation of free and bound labels is required and a homogeneous assay can be achieved.

A partial list of the indicators which have been employed as immunochemical labels is found in Table I. The methods are listed in the table in the order they will be discussed in the text.

Table I

IMMUNOCHEMICAL LABELS

1. Radioisotopes
2. Free Radicals
3. Fluorescent Molecules
4. Chemiluminescent Molecules
5. Enzyme Cofactors
6. Enzymes

EMIT® and FRAT® are registered trademarks of the Syva Company, Palo Alto, California.

2. Radioisotopes

The familiar method of radioimmunoassay (RIA), which uses radioisotopes as labels, was first developed in 1960 by Yalow and Berson. RIA is indoubtedly the immunoassay method in widest use (Parker, 1976). Commonly used radionuclides are the β-emitters ^3H, ^{14}C and the γ-emitter ^{125}I. The principal advantage of RIA is the sensitivity achievable by use of high specific activity labeled materials. However, there are some serious disadvantages with the method, including the requirement that free and bound labels be separated, health hazards, disposal of radioisotopes, expense of counters, and limited life of reagents labeled with ^{125}I. For this nuclide, the usable lifetime of most reagents is less than two months.

Soon after the significance of RIA was recognized, efforts commenced in laboratories around the world to develop quantitative non-isotopic immunoassays which did not require separation steps. During the past ten years, these efforts have resulted in the development of a variety of homogeneous methods which employ the alternate labels listed in Table I. Any of the labels listed in Table I can also be employed in a heterogeneous assay mode; the emphasis here will be placed on the homogeneous methods.

3. Free Radicals

Free radicals have been used in a method known as FRAT®—Free Radical Assay Technique—initially described by Leute, Ullman, Goldstein, and Herzenberg in 1971 (Leute *et al*, 1972). They used stable nitroxide free radicals to spin-label the drug morphine. Since the properties of free radicals, as observed by their electron spin resonance (esr) spectra, are very sensitive to environment and molecular motion, the signals of free and antibody-bound spin-labeled drugs are different. The modulation of the esr signal by the antibody-antigen reaction formed the basis of a homogeneous assay method. FRAT® assays were marketed briefly by Syva Company as the first commercial homogeneous non-isotopic immunoassays. Their main limitations were the complexity of esr instrumentation and lack of availability of such instrumentation in clinical laboratories.

4. Fluorescent Molecules

Fluorescence immunoassays had their origins in the fluorescent antibody techniques for histochemical localization of antigens developed in the late 1950's and early 1960's (Goldman, 1968; Nairn, 1976). A discussion of several types of homogeneous immunoassays which rely on a modulation of the fluorescence properties of a labeled antigen follows.

A. Fluorescence Polarization Assays

The principle of fluorescence polarization (FP) was first applied to immunoassay by Dandliker and coworkers (1964; 1973). The FP of a small fluorescent-labeled molecule tumbling freely in solution is very low. However, when the labeled molecule becomes complexed with antibody, its molecular motion is slowed and the FP increases. This modulation phenomenon provides the means to distinguish between free and bound labels. Recently Landon *et al* have described routine FP assay for the drugs gentamicin and phenytoin in human serum (Watson *et al*, 1976; McGregor *et al*, 1978).

B. Fluorescence Quenching or Enhancement Assay

The effects of protein binding on the fluorescence properties of small molecules have been exploited for some time in biophysical studies of proteins (Stryer, 1968; Edelman and McClure,

1968). Assays for gentamicin and thyroxine based on the quenching or enhancement of fluorescence intensity of the labeled antigen have recently been reported (Shaw et al, 1977; Smith, 1977). At present, it is difficult to predict the generality and applicability of these methods.

C. Fluorescence Excitation Transfer Assay

Ullman, Schwarzberg, and Rubenstein (1976) have described a novel immunoassay technique which uses the principle of fluorescence excitation transfer to detect antibody-antigen complex formation. Several assay modes can be employed. Of most interest, for measurement of low molecular weight drugs, is the mode which uses an antigen labeled with a fluorescent chromophore, acting as an energy donor, and an antibody labeled with a second chromophore, acting as an energy acceptor or quencher. Since excitation energy transfer is distance dependent, transfer occurs only in the complex between labeled components. Therefore, no separation of reactants is required. Assays were described for opiates and for human IgG (Ullman et al, 1976).

D. Reactant-labeled Fluorescence Assays

Burd and his coworkers have described a homogeneous assay which uses a drug labeled with fluorescent dye (1977). The drug-dye conjugate is a substrate for an enzyme which is added to the assay mixture. The enzyme catalyzes a reaction which results in a change in the fluorescence properties of the drug-dye conjugate. The reaction of antibody with the conjugate reduces the amount of substrate available for enzymatic conversion. The measured fluorescence is proportional to the amount of drug in the sample. A clinical assay of this type for the drug gentamicin has been reported (Burd et al, 1977).

5. Chemiluminescent Molecules

Schroeder et al have described the use of luminol derivatives as labels in competitive immunoassays in which the chemiluminescence of the free labeled antigen is generated by an enzymatic reaction (1976; 1977). This method is a variant of the reactant-labeled fluorescence assay.

6. Enzyme Cofactors

The enzyme cofactors NAD and ATP have also been reported as labels in another variant of the reactant-labeled immunoassay (Carrico et al, 1976a; Schroeder et al, 1976; Carrico et al, 1976b). Enzymatic activity can be detected using either spectrophotometry or luminescence measurements. When luminescence detection is used, the product of the initial enzymatic reaction is fed into an enzyme system which catalyzes the production of light.

7. Enzymes

Enzymes, the most frequently used non-isotopic labels, have been employed in both heterogeneous and homogeneous assay modes. Since the work on heterogeneous enzyme immunoassay has been frequently reviewed (Schuurs and Van Weemen, 1977; Scharpe et al, 1976; Wisdom, 1976), the only method to be considered here is the EMIT® homogeneous enzyme immunoassay technique (Rubenstein et al, 1972; Rubenstein, 1978).

8. Homogeneous Enzyme Immunoassay

The principle of an EMIT® drug assay is depicted in Figure 1. The method employs an enzyme as the label for a drug. A drug derivative is attached to

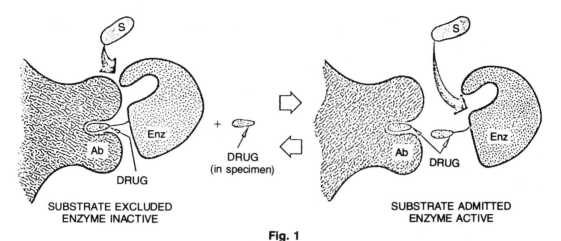

Fig. 1

SCHEMATIC REPRESENTATION OF THE EMIT® HOMOGENEOUS ENZYME
IMMUNOASSAY FOR DRUG DETERMINATION.

the enzyme to form an enzyme-drug conjugate. The activity of this enzyme-drug conjugate is modulated when anti-drug antibody binds to the conjugate. When the sample (usually a body fluid) is mixed with the antibody and the enzyme-labeled drug, free drug molecules in the sample compete with the enzyme-labeled molecules for a limited number of antibody binding sites. The more free drug in the sample, the more enzyme remains unbound. Enzyme activity can be directly correlated with the concentration of drug in the specimen. Figure 1 shows a representation of inhibition of activity and the mechanism of this inhibition is described as a steric exclusion of the substrate. This concept adequately describes the mechanism when the enzyme lysozyme is used (Rubenstein *et al*, 1972; Schneider *et al*, 1973). However, when malate dehydrogenase and glucose-6-phosphate dehydrogenase (G-6-PDH) are employed, enzyme conformational change has been implicated as the mechanism of activity modulation (Rowley *et al*, 1975; 1976).

Because enzymes are biochemical amplifiers, the EMIT® technique has potential for a very high level of sensitivity. The sensitivity depends on many factors, among them the choice of enzyme, length of incubation, and method for de-tection of catalytic activity. The sensitivity limit of current EMIT® assays is in the ng/ml range.

The EMIT® assay procedure is straightforward. The sample, plus anti-body/substrate, and enzyme-drug conjugate are measured and mixed using an automatic pipetter-diluter. The assay mixture is then aspirated into the flow cell of a standard laboratory spectrophotometer. The kinetic determination of enzyme activity requires thirty seconds, and a single assay is completed in one minute.

Qualitative assays of this type have been developed for detection of drugs of abuse in urine. Assays for opiates, barbiturates, amphetamines, benzodiazepines, and benzoyl ecgonine (cocaine metabolite) (Schneider *et al*, 1973; Brattin and Sunshine, 1974; Mule *et al*, 1974) which employ lysozyme as the enzyme label are currently available, and assays for phencyclidine (PCP) and tetrahydrocannabinol (THC) (Rodgers *et al*, 1978) are under development.

Quantitative assays using G-6-PDH as an enzyme label have been developed for a wide variety of therapeutic drugs. G-6-PDH catalyzes the conversion of D-glucose-6-phosphate to D-gluconolacetone-6-phosphate with the concommitant reduction of NAD to NADH. The use of a bacterial enzyme rather than enzyme from a mammalian source reduces endogenous sample interference, and a serum pretreatment step is not required.

The value of a knowledge of the serum concentration of a therapeutic drug is becoming increasingly recognized, particularly when toxic effects occur above a very narrow therapeutic range. Assays have been developed for a wide variety of therapeutic control agents (TCA). A list of these is shown in Table II.

The procedure in all of the TCA assays is similar. They employ a spectrophotometer with a thermally regulated flow cell, a timer-printer which times the data collection and calculates the rate of enzyme activity, and an automatic pipetter-diluter by which all additions are made.

The $50\mu l$ serum sample is diluted

Table II

ASSAYS FOR DRUGS OF THERAPEUTIC CONTROL (TCA) IN SERUM

Reference	Antiepileptic Drugs	Therapeutic Concentration Range (μg/ml)	Assay Range
Pippenger et al, 1975; Bastiani et al, 1978	Phenytoin	10 - 20	2.5 - 30
Pippenger et al, 1975; Bastiani et al, 1978	Phenobarbital	15 - 40	5.0 - 80
Pippenger et al, 1975; Bastiani et al, 1978	Primidone	5 - 12	2.5 - 20
Pippenger et al, 1975; Bastiani et al, 1978	Carbamazepine	4 - 12	2.0 - 20
Pippenger et al, 1975; Bastiani et al, 1978	Ethosuximide	40 - 100	10.0 - 150
	Cardioactive Drugs		
Chang et al, 1975	Digoxin	1 - 2 ng/ml	0.5 - 8.0 ng/ml
Cobb et al, 1975	Lidocaine	2 - 5	1.0 - 12
Fanciullo et al, 1978	Procainamide	4 - 8	1.0 - 16
Izutsu et al, 1978	N-acetylprocainamide	4 - 8	1.0 - 16
Chegwidden et al, 1978	Propranolol*	50 - 200 ng/ml	25 - 400 ng/ml
	Quinidine*	2 - 6	0.5 - 8.0
	Respiratory Agents		
Chang and Bastiani, 1977	Theophylline	10 - 20	2.5 - 40
	Chemotherapy Drugs		
Gushaw et al, 1978	Methotrexate	-	50 ng/ml - 500 μg/ml
	Antibacterial Drugs		
Kabakoff et al, 1978	Gentamicin*	4 - 12	1 - 16
	Tobramyacin*		1 - 16
	Amikacin*		
	Antidepressant Drugs		
	Imipramine*		
	Desimipramine*		
	Amitriptyline*		
	Nortriptyline*		

*Currently under development

twice with 250μl of assay buffer followed by addition of antibody. This solution is incubated for a few seconds before addition of enzyme conjugate. At the high concentration of reagents employed, the system is analogous to sequential addition in RIA, where the later addition of label to preincubated sample and antibody results in a more sensitive assay. Thus, as binding is instantaneous, a state of equilibrium between antibody-bound and free enzyme conjugate has been achieved by the time the enzyme rate is measured.

A standard curve is obtained by plotting the change of absorbance over 30 seconds against the concentration of standard. A linear response is obtained when the logarithmic concentration of the drug (in μg/ml) is plotted on the horizontal axis, and the vertical axis is a refined logit function of the enzyme rate. This transforms the typically sigmoidal immunoassay standard curve to a straight line, and leads to more precise data interpretation. The system is stable; a standard curve is useful for at least one working day.

9. Anticonvulsant Drugs (AED)

A summary of field performance data for the AED assays (Bastiani and Chang, 1978) is given in Tables III, IV, and V on this page and on the opposite page.

a) PRECISION of the EMIT® assay system was determined by replicate analysis of a serum based calibrator. Coefficients of Variation (C.V.) which were obtained by individual investigators were:

Table III

	Coefficients of Variation
Phenytoin (10.0 μg/ml)	9.1%, 4.8%, 5.7%
Phenobarbital (20.0 μg/ml)	6.8%, 3.8%, 5.2%
Primidone (10.0 μg/ml)	6.4%, 3.3%, 5.1%
Carbamazepine (5.0 μg/ml)	5.5%, 3.8%, 3.9%, 4.7%
Ethosuximide (50.0 μg/ml)	11.1%, 11.8%, 9.7%, 11.3%

In summary, the precision of the EMIT® Phenytoin, Phenobarbital, Primidone and Carbamazepine Assays averages between a C.V. of 5-6%. The Ethosuximide Assay is less precise, with an average C.V. of 11%.

b) ACCURACY was assessed by analysis of a set of unknown spiked samples (Table IV). The correlation statistics of spiked versus EMIT® mean assayed values were:

Table IV

	Correlation Coefficient	Standard Error of the Estimate	Regression Line Slope	Y-Intercept
Phenytoin	0.995	0.65 μg/ml	1.04	−0.21 μg/ml
Phenobarbital	0.980	3.19 μg/ml	0.89	+1.48 μg/ml
Primidone	0.995	0.49 μg/ml	0.99	+0.14 μg/ml
Carbamazepine	0.998	0.24 μg/ml	1.08	−0.26 μg/ml
Ethosuximide	0.997	1.88 μg/ml	1.01	−3.56 μg/ml

c) SPECIFICITY

There is no significant crossreactivity among the five EMIT® AED Assays. In addition, metabolites of these five drugs have not been shown to crossreact to a clinically significant degree.

A partial list of metabolite crossreactivities which was derived from the study of representative reagent lots is as follows (The quantities listed are the amounts necessary to cause a 30% error in the quantitation of the middle calibrator in each of the respective assays.):

Phenytoin Assay—5-(p-hydroxyphenyl)-5-phenylhydantoin crossreacts at 18 μg/ml; *Primidone*—2-phenyl-2-ethyl-malondiamide crossreacts at >500 μg/ml; *Carbamazepine Assay*—Carbamazepine-10, 11-epoxide crossreacts at 14 μg/ml, Iminostilbene crossreacts at 34 μg/ml.

The AED Assay series show no clinically significant response to other medications common to epileptic patients.

d) COMPARATIVE ANALYSIS (Table V)

Comparison of the EMIT® Assay System with gas liquid chromatography (GLC) was performed on serum specimens from patients on antiepileptic drug therapy.

Table V

	Phenytoin	Phenobarbital	Primidone	Carbamazepine	Ethosuximide
Number of Samples	717	502	178	305	265
Correlation Coefficient	0.94	0.94	0.96	0.95	0.95
Mean					
EMIT® (μg/ml)	13.03	23.33	10.70	5.27	52.98
GLC (μg/ml)	13.40	24.70	10.71	5.37	52.33
Mean Difference (μg/ml)	0.37	1.37	0.01	0.10	−0.56

The determination of phenobarbital by GLC is dependent upon the internal standard used. Valid results were obtained only when p-tolylphenobarbital was used as the internal standard.

The advantage of these assays over existing high-pressure liquid chromatography and GLC methods is the speed with which a result is obtained, meaning that a patient's sample may be assayed during his or her visit to a clinician and the dose of drug adjusted accordingly. In pediatric epilepsy in particular, repeated monitoring of serum concentrations by GLC, requiring 1ml of serum, is difficult. Using the EMIT® assays, a 50μl sample volume is sufficient for five determinations.

The potential application of these assays to determine salivary concentrations of the drugs, which have been shown to correlate with serum concentrations, presents an interesting non-invasive methodology for use in pediatric practice.

10. Cardioactive Drugs (CAD)

A list of EMIT® assays for CAD is given in Table II. With the exception of the assay for digoxin, all are performed following the protocol previously described for the anti-epileptic and drug abuse assays.

Since the RIA for digoxin was first described in 1969, the clinical benefit derived from a knowledge of the serum concentration of this drug has led to an increased demand for the assay. Due to its presence in serum at concentrations in the nanomole per liter range, the sensitivity requirement imposes a longer read time on the enzyme assay. In the batch procedure, 60 determinations may be made in 90 minutes, where tubes are incubated for 30 minutes at 30°C between the first and second absorbance readings. The method is precise and correlates with RIA (r = 0.98). The test is readily automated by adaption to centrifugal analyzers and to the ABA-100 (Scoggin et al, 1978).

11. Theophylline

Recent developments in the clinical pharmacology of theophylline have resulted in a renewed emphasis and improved use of this drug in the treatment of asthma. Today, theophylline is considered the primary drug of choice in the treatment and prevention of asthmatic symptoms in children and adults. The relationship between theophylline dosage and the likelihood of achieving both therapeutic effect and toxicity has been reported. However, because there are remarkable variations in the rates of individual metabolism of theophylline in both children and adults, large percentages of patients in any population receiving the useful dosage will either not achieve a therapeutic effect or be at risk of toxicity. This is particularly true in the case of young infants as they are very susceptible to seizure, while other adverse side effects are usually difficult to recognize.

Figure 2 is a diagram indicating the

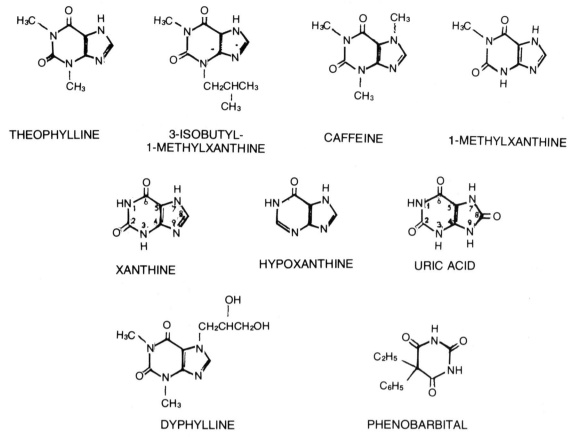

Fig. 2

THEOPHYLLINE AND RELATED STRUCTURES

variety of structurally-related substances that are important in an assay for theophylline. Variations in the alkyl substituents on the nitrogen atoms provide a dazzling array of substituted xanthines and hypoxanthines for consideration. In order for an assay to be widely useful, the antisera must differentiate theophylline from caffeine, theobromine, and other common xanthine derivatives. In the EMIT® theophylline assay, 3-isobutyl-1-methylxanthine is recognized approximately as well as theophylline by the antisera. This is not unexpected since the 3-position of the xanthine ring was used as the position for conjugation to the protein carrier. 1-methyl-xanthine, 8-chlorotheophylline, and caffeine have shown very little crossreactivity in this assay. This is important since caf-

feine is found in soft drinks, coffee, and chocolate, making it one of the most commonly found stimulants in our diet. 1-methyl-xanthine is a common inactive metabolite of theophylline and caffeine, and 8-chlorotheophylline is used in motion sickness medication.

Potential interfering substances were studied by adding various concentrations of each compound to pooled human serum to determine the concentration necessary to give an error in assay quantitation. Such an error is defined as the concentration of cross-reactant necessary to produce a 30% quantitation error in a human serum containing $10.0\mu g/ml$ of theophylline, i.e. elevation of the analytical value to $13.0\mu g/ml$. The compounds studied in this manner are listed in Table VI.

Table VI

CONCENTRATION OF A CROSSREACTANT Necessary to Produce a 30% Quantitation Error in a Sample Containing 10 μg/ml Theophylline

Caffeine (1,3,7-trimethylxanthine)	> 75 μg/ml
Theobromine (3,7-dimethylxanthine)	> 150 μg/ml
Paraxanthine (1,7-dimethylxanthine)	> 100 μg/ml
1-methylxanthine	> 20 μg/ml
3-methylxanthine	> 150 μg/ml
7-methylxanthine	> 100 μg/ml
Xanthine	> 200 μg/ml
Hypoxanthine	> 300 μg/ml
1,3-dimethyluric acid	> 150 μg/ml
1,3,7-trimethyluric acid	> 200 μg/ml
1-methyluric acid	> 200 μg/ml
Uric acid	> 200 μg/ml
Dyphylline (7-dihydroxypropyl-theophylline)	> 400 μg/ml
Urea	>1000 μg/ml
8-chlorotheophylline	> 50 μg/ml
Phenobarbital	> 150 μg/ml

Table VII

CORRELATION STATISTICS—Comparative Analysis of Theophylline Patient Samples

	HPLC				UV Spectrophotometry		
	Lab 1	Lab 2	Lab 3	Lab 4	Lab 5	Lab 6	Lab 7
Number of Samples	101	90	112	100	102	85	96
Correlation Coefficient	0.98	0.97	0.95	0.95	0.87	0.86	0.97
Mean (μg/ml)							
EMIT®	12.16	14.69	13.22	8.01	9.25	15.23	13.30
HPLC or UV	11.45	15.80	12.67	7.75	8.45	16.02	11.37

The protocol for the assay is the same as described previously for the AED assays. The assay has been found accurate and precise (Chang and Bastiani, 1977) and has recently been described in detail (Rubenstein, 1978; Gushaw et al, 1977). Data from both the EMIT® assay and a reference method (HPLC, UV) were analyzed (Table VII). No significant difference in the results has been observed, thereby giving support to the postulate that metabolites or drugs with similar structure do not interfere with the EMIT® theophylline assay. A scattergram (Figure 3) has been prepared by plotting the data obtained from one of the field sites.

12. Methotrexate

Methotrexate, a folic acid antagonist, has been in clinical use for over 20 years. Prior to 1967, it was used in comparatively small doses in the treatment of acute leukemia and diseases such as severe psoriasis. Considerable clinical experience with high-dose methotrexate regimens in treating a variety of neoplastic diseases has been gained during the

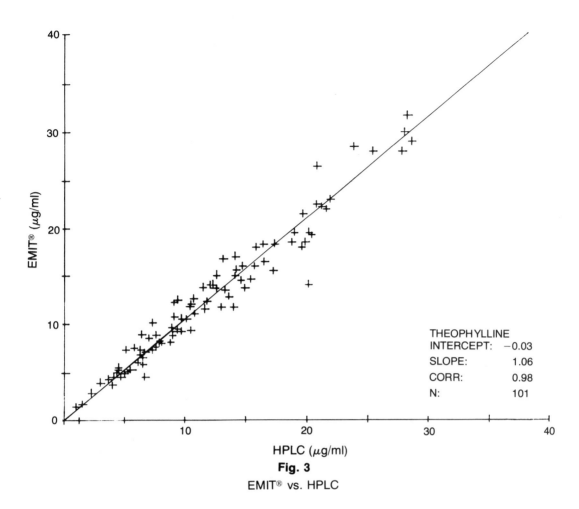

Fig. 3
EMIT® vs. HPLC

past decade, supporting the hypothesis that saturation of certain neoplastic cells with the drug could elicit an effect which was not obtainable with lower doses. High-dose methotrexate therapy has become common in the management of acute carcinoma.

Routine monitoring of plasma methotrexate concentrations permits early recognition of patients at risk of developing serious toxicity. Depending on the drug regimen, peak serum methotrexate concentrations may reach 10^{-2} to 10^{-5} moles/liter. The EMIT® methotrexate assay (Gushaw and Miller, 1978) enables laboratories to conveniently measure serum concentrations within a few minutes of receipt of the sample. The assay is sensitive to serum drug concentrations between 2×10^{-7} and 2.6×10^{-3} moles/liter,

a range corresponding to values observed in high-dose therapy. No clinically significant crossreactivity has been observed from compounds related to or concurrently administered with methotrexate. Additionally, the method is compatible with most existing instrumentation used in enzyme activity measurements. A scattergram analysis of samples obtained from patients on methotrexate therapy is shown in Figure 4. This figure is a comparison of results obtained by the EMIT® methotrexate assay and those obtained by a radioimmunoassay (Paxton and Rowell, 1977) and an enzymatic assay (Falk *et al*, 1976) for methotrexate. Since the drug concentration of interest spans four orders of magnitude, logarithmic axes are used in Figure 4.

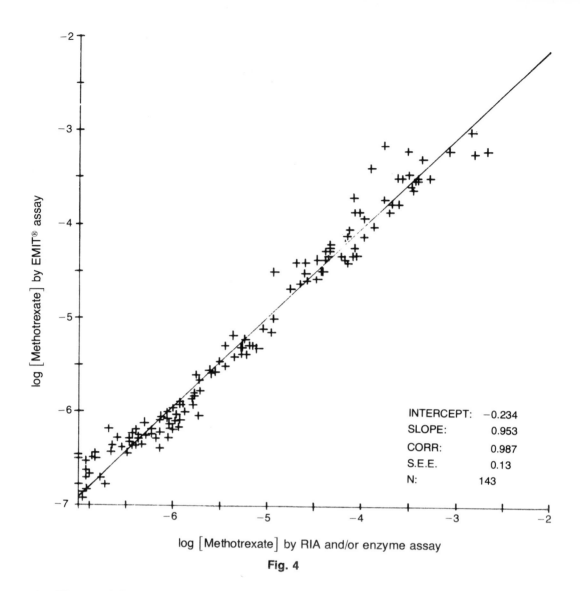

log [Methotrexate] by RIA and/or enzyme assay

Fig. 4

13. Thyroid Function Assays

The thyroid hormones are important regulators of body metabolism. Their presence is critical to growth, development, and maintenance of good health. So important are these hormones that abnormal levels at any age can produce mental and physical disabilities. In newborns, for example, undetected thyroid deficiency can cause irreparable mental retardation and physical deformity. With the recognition of the importance of thyroid hormones to good health and the difficulty in differentiating between thyroid disease and other illnesses, tests to confirm or rule out this endocrine problem are usually included in an initial diagnostic workup. Today, clinicians consider blood level measurements of these hormones important diagnostic tools. As thyroid testing methods become easier and less expensive, many laboratories will no doubt add thyroid tests to traditional biochemical screens or organ profiles.

A progression of methodologies has been used to monitor thyroid functions by measurements of thyroxine. Historically, the most important procedures begin with the measurement of protein-bound iodine. This analysis was performed in the clinical chemistry lab due to the procedural requirements of the test. This initial method was replaced by the more sensitive radioassays involving competitive protein binding. The procedure described by Murphy and Patee allowed the relatively specific measurement of thyroxine. Interestingly, the radiolabel employed in the method resulted in the migration of the test from the clinical chemistry laboratory to the nuclear medicine area. The movement was enhanced by the introduction of sensitive radioimmunoassays using specific antithyroxine antibodies.

Recently, EMIT® thyroxine assays have been introduced to accommodate existing single (Jaklitsch *et al*, 1976) and multichannel enzyme analyzers (Galen and Forman, 1977; Besemer and Chandler, 1977; McReynolds *et al*, 1977). With this innovation, thyroxine assays can once again be performed in the clinical laboratory. More important, existing automated analyzers can be employed to perform T-4 determinations by the same technicians who currently carry out enzyme and blood chemistry tests.

A variety of EMIT® thyroxine assay systems is listed in Table VIII with various performance characteristics. All systems result in coefficients of variation of less than 10% with equivalent quantitation and normal range values. Correlation between the EMIT® ABA thyroxine and a commercial RIA thyroxine kit is presented in Figure 5.

The manual assay is performed in batches containing up to 60 samples. A sample throughput of 40-60 samples per hour makes this test useful for smaller hospitals and clinics that do not have high workload, and, therefore, do not require faster throughput and less technician involvement. The ABA-100 or Centrifugal Analyzer T-4 assays allow hundreds of samples to be analyzed per day, making these systems applicable for larger clinical laboratories or for screening applications. Of course, incorporation of the T-4 test into the domain of multichannel analyzers makes the possibility of screening patients for thyroid abnormality quite intriguing.

14. Automation

The homogeneous property of EMIT® assays renders these techniques readily applicable to automated systems. This permits immunoassays to be performed on many automated enzyme analyzers, both single and multichannel.

Table VIII
EMIT® THYROXINE ASSAYS

	ABA-100	Centrifichem®	Manual	Autochemist
Sample volume, μ[1]	20	25	50	75
Total assay time, min[1]	45	30	45	—
Technician time, min[1]	20	15	20	—
Potential throughput assay/hr	80-100	100-150	50	180
Reagent stability				
Lyophilized	1 year	1 year	1 year	—
Reconstituted	4 months	4 months	4 months	6 months

[1]Batch of 28-30 assays.
Precision—less than 8% coefficient of variation (μg/dl)
Accuracy—comparison of RIA methods give correlation coefficients of 0.92-0.96.
Specificity—no known clinically significant
cross-reactants: minimal interference from crossly abnormal serum specimens (hemolysis, lipemia, icterus)

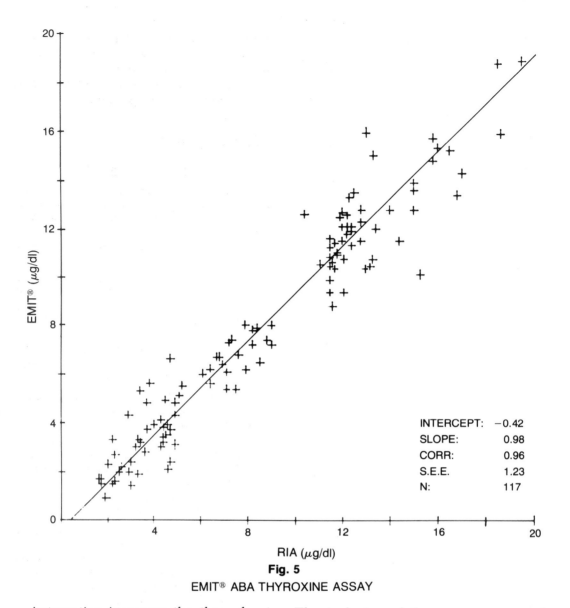

Fig. 5

EMIT® ABA THYROXINE ASSAY

Automation increases the throughput of the assay, reduces technician time and fatigue, and with automated data handling, reduces transcription errors. Assay precision is improved on these systems as manual pipetting is reduced. However, precision has also been found to depend on the accuracy of temperature control in the instrument.

While it may be difficult to justify the requirement for an automated digoxin assay except in large reference labs, perhaps the most important need for automation involves the thyroid assays.

The inclusion of these assays on multichannel biochemistry profiling instruments enables laboratories to perform them with other routine analyses without splitting the sample and without the potential of delay in reporting the result or error in data transcription.

15. Conclusion

Much has been made of the relative arguments for and against RIA versus EIA (Anon., 1976; Ekins, 1976), in particular, the relative stability of reagents, safety, and cost of equipment. There is no question that enzyme labels have a longer shelf life than ^{125}I-labeled compounds, the radioisotope most commonly used in RIA today. The health hazard depends entirely on the quantity of isotope being handled, although its disposal presents an increasing environmental problem. The most ambiguous factor is the equipment cost. If an enzyme analyzer were not present where an automated gamma counter already existed, it would be expensive to change to an EMIT® system. However, with the increasing demand for RIA's, laboratories are finding that available counting time is taken up. Transferring such assays as T-4 and digoxin to enzyme analyzers frees counting time for the more esoteric RIA's which require high sensitivity and cannot yet be replaced by non-isotopic techniques.

The future for enzyme immunoassays seems bright. In the past few years, these techniques have been increasingly applied to clinical diagnosis and treatment. Further developments aimed at improved separation procedures and in heterogeneous assay sensitivity will make these techniques increasingly applicable to clinical laboratories around the world. The EMIT® technique is the prime example of both a homogeneous and a non-isotopic immunoassay. Being highly versatile, the technique has already had significant impact on two areas of diagnostic medicine: measurement of drugs of abuse and therapeutic drug monitoring. The fluorescence and reactant-labeled methods discussed in this paper have not yet been widely applied, but appear to hold promise in expanding the analytical capabilities of clinical chemists. The main thrust of the intense activity in the immunoassay area has been in the development of clinical diagnostic procedures. However, it is easily appreciated that immunochemical assays have potential in areas such as industrial quality and process control, environmental analysis, and forensic analysis. Significant advances in the application of immunoassay techniques in these new areas are predicted.

16. References

Anonymous (1976). *Lancet* **2**, 406

Bastiani, R. J. and Chang, J. (1978). "Summary Report: Performance Evaluation of the EMIT® AED Assays," Syva Co., Palo Alto, California

Besemer, D. M. and Chandler, J. R. (1977). *Clin Chem* **23**, 1083

Brattin, W. J. and Sunshine, I. (1974). *In* "Immunoassays for Drugs Subject to Abuse" (Mule, S. J., Sunshine, I., Braude, M. and Willette, R. E., eds.) pp. 107-116, CRC Press, Cleveland

Burd, J. F., Wong, R. C., Feeney, J. E., Carrico, R. J. and Boguslaski, R. C. (1977). *Clin Chem* **23**, 1402-08

Carrico, R. J., Christner, J. E., Boguslaski, R. C. and Yeung, K. K. (1976a). *Analytical Biochemistry* **72**, 283-292

Carrico, R. J., Yeung, K. K., Schroeder, H. R., Boguslaski, R. C., Buckler, R. T. and Christner, J. E. (1976b). *Analytical Biochemistry* **76**, 95-110

Chang, J. J., Crowl, C. P. and Schneider, R. S. (1975). *Clin Chem* **21**, 967

Chang, J. Y. and Bastiani, R. J. (1977). "Clinical Study No. 41., Summary Report: Performance Evaluation of the EMIT® Theophylline Assay," Syva Co., Palo Alto, California

Chegwidden, K., Pirio, M. R., Singh, P., Gushaw, J. B., Miller, J. G. and Schneider, R. S. (1978). *Clin Chem* **24**, 1056

Cobb, M. E., Buckley, N., Hu, M. W., Miller, J. G., Singh, P. and Schneider, R. S. (1975). *Clin Chem* **21**, 967

Cohen, R. J. and Benedek, G. B. (1975). *Immunochem* **12**, 249-351

Dandliker, W. B., Kelly, R. J., Dandliker, J., Farguhar, J. and Levin, J. (1973). *Immunochem* **10**, 219

Dandliker, W. B., Schapiro, H. C., Meduski, J. W., Alonso, R., Feigen, G. H. and Hamrick, J. R., Jr. (1964). *Immunochem* **1**, 165

Edelman, G. M. and McClure, W. O. (1968). *Accounts of Chemical Research 1* **3**, 65-70

Ekins, R. (1976). *Lancet* **2**, 569 (letter)

Falk, L. C., Clark, D. R., Kalman, S. M. and Long, T. F. (1976). *Clin Chem* **22**, 785

Fanciullo, R. A., Huber, N., Izutsu, A., Pirio, M. R., Buckley, N., Singh, P., Gushaw, J. B., Miller, J. G. and Schneider, R. S. (1978). *Clin Chem* **24**, 1056

Galen, R. S. and Forman, D. W. (1977). *Clin Chem* **23**, 119

Goldman, M. (1968). "Fluorescent Antibody Methods," Academic Press, New York

Gushaw, J. B., Hu, M. W., Singh, P., Miller, J. G. and Schneider, R. S. (1977). *Clin Chem* **23**, 1144

Gushaw, J. B. and Miller, J. G. (1978). *Clin Chem* **24**, 1032

Izutsu, A., Pirio, M. R., Buckley, N., Singh, P., Gushaw, J. B., Miller, J. G. and Schneider, R. S. (1978). *Clin Chem* **24**, 1055

Jaklitsch, A. P., Schneider, R. S., Johannes, R. J., Levine, J. E. and Rosenberg, G. L. (1976). *Clin Chem* **22**, 1185

Kabakoff, D. S., Leung, D. and Singh, P. (1978). *Clin Chem* **24**, 1055

Leute, R. K., Ullman, E. F., Goldstein, A. and Herzenberg, L. A. (1971). *Nature* **236**, 253

Leute, R. K., Ullman, E. F. and Goldstein, A. (1972). *J Amer Med Soc* **221**, 1231

McGregor, A. R., Crookall-Greening, J. O., Landon, J. and Smith, D. S. (1978). *Clin Chim Acta* **83**, 161-66

McReynolds, C. W., Schoder, S. M. and Schneider, R. S. (1977). *Clin Chem* **23**, 1123

Mule, S. J., Bastos, M. L. and Jukafsky, D. (1974). *Clin Chem* **20**, 243-48

Nairn, R. C. (1976). "Fluorescent Protein Tracing," 4th ed., Churchill Livingstone, Edinburgh, Scotland

Parker, C. W. (1976). "Radioimmunoassay of Biologically Active Compounds," Prentice-Hall, Englewood Cliffs, New Jersey

Paxton, J. W. and Rowell, F. J. (1977). *Clin Chim Acta* **80**, 563

Peetoom, F. (1971). *Am J Med Tech* **37** 12, 1-14

Pippenger, C. E., Bastiani, R. J. and Schneider, R. S. (1975). *In* "Clinical Pharmacology of Antiepileptic Drugs" (Schneider, H., Janz, D., Gardner-Thorpe, C., Meinardi,

H. and Sherwin, A. L., eds.) pp. 331-36, Springer-Verlag, New York

Rodgers, R., Crowl, C. P., Eimstad, W. M., Hu, M. W., Kam, J. K., Ronald, R. C., Rowley, G. L. and Ullman, E. F. (1978). *Clin Chem* **24**, 95-100

Rowley, G. L., Rubenstein, K. E., Huisjen, J. and Ullman, E. F. (1975). *J Biol Chem* **250**, 2759-3766

Rowley, G. L., Rubenstein, K. E., Weber, S. T. and Ullman, E. F. (1976). *In* "Abstracts of the 172nd American Chemical Society National Meeting," Biological Chemistry Section, Abstract No. 151, San Francisco

Rubenstein, K. E. (1978). *Scand J Immuno* **8**, Suppl. 7, 57-62

Rubenstein, K. E., Schneider, R. S. and Ullman, E. F. (1972). *Biochem Biophys Res Comm* **47**, 846-51

Scharpe, S. L., Cooreman, W. M., Blomme, W. J. and Lackeman, G. M. (1976). *Clin Chem* **22**, 733-38

Schneider, R. S., Lindquist, P., Wong, E. T., Rubenstein, K. E. and Ullman, E. F. (1973). *Clin Chem* **19**, 821-25

Schroeder, H. R., Carrico, R. J., Boguslaski, R. C. and Christner, J. E. (1976). *Analytical Biochemistry* **72**, 283-92

Schroeder, H. R., Vogelhut, P. O., Carrico, R. J., Boguslaski, R. C. and Buckler, R. T. (1976). *Analytical Chem* **48**, 1933-37

Schroeder, H. R., Yeager, F. M., Boguslaski, R. C., Snoke, E. O. and Buckler, R. T. (1977). *Clin Chem* **23**, 1123

Schuurs, A. H. W. M. and Van Weemen, B. K. (1977). *Clin Chim Acta* **81**, 1-40

Scoggin, D., Petrehn, J. and Besemer, D. (1978). *Clin Chem* **24**, 1055

Shaw, E. J., Watson, R. A. A., Landon, J. and Smith, D. S. (1977). *J Clin Path* **30**, 526-31

Smith, D. S. (1977). *FEBS Letters* **77**, 25-27

Stryer, L. (1968). *Science* **162**, 526-33

Ullman, E. F., Schwarzberg, M. and Rubenstein, D. E. (1976). *J Biol Chem* **251**, 4172-78

Watson, R. A. A., Landon, J., Shaw, E. J. and Smith, D. S. (1976). *Clin Chim Acta* **73**, 51-55

Wisdom, G. B. (1976). *Clin Chem* **22**, 1243-55

Yalow, R. S. and Berson, S. A. (1960). *J Clin Invest* **39**, 1157-75

CHAPTER **II**

Status of Solid-Phase Enzyme Immunoassays

G. C. SAUNDERS, V.M.D.

Table of Contents

1. Introduction

Solid-phase (or heterogeneous) enzyme immunoassays (EIA's) for a variety of antibodies, antigens, and haptens are being developed at a very rapid rate. Because of their basic simplicity, sensitivity, and accuracy, at least in this writer's view, they will probably replace many of the common types of immunoassays currently in use. That is, such fun-to-do procedures as complement fixation, hemagglutination, hemagglutination inhibition, and immunoprecipitation may become classroom curiosities. Indeed, even immunofluorescent and radioimmunoassays soon should be gradually replaced by solid-phase EIA's, as is already occurring with homogeneous EIA's in the hapten area.

Why are solid-phase EIA's becoming so popular? Their attributes can be listed as follows: (1) they are primary binding assays and do not require the participation of secondary events (e.g., complement fixation, agglutination, etc.) to obtain a readable result; (2) solid-phase EIA's are technically easy to perform as they employ simple incubation and wash protocols; (3) the enzyme conjugates are stable for prolonged periods (usually indefinitely) and are relatively inexpensive; (4) the versatility of the assays ranges from quick antibody screening tests to very sensitive, quantitative assays of haptens; (5) test results can be read with simple, inexpensive colorimeters or spectrophotometers; (6) the simplicity, sensitivity, and lack of a need for expensive isotope counting equipment allow these assays to be performed in small, community-type hospitals; and (7) when necessary, the methodology can be easily automated.

The remainder of this chapter will describe the principles and applications of the major types of solid-phase EIA's now in use. In addition, some operational considerations and a discussion of the "art" of performing these assays will be included. Finally, a brief description of an available automated EIA system will be given. The recent excellent review by Schuurs and Van Weemen (1977) is recommended to readers who require more information concerning specific assay parameters.

Description and Applications of Solid-Phase Enzyme Immunoassays

A. Indirect Solid-Phase Enzyme Immunoassay

Indirect solid-phase EIA's are most often used to detect serum antibody to antigens derived from infectious and parasitic disease agents. The binding sequence for an indirect solid-phase EIA is illustrated in Figure 1. Antigen is first bound to the solid phase (e.g., 96-well microplate); this is usually accomplished by simple adsorption using a special adsorption buffer (see Table I). Suspect serum is then incubated with the antigen, and if the serum contains antibody, it will bind to the adsorbed antigen as illustrated (Figure 1). The incubation time varies with the assay, but ranges from just a few minutes to several hours. After incubation, nonbound serum is removed by several washes, and then enzyme-labeled antispecies antibody is

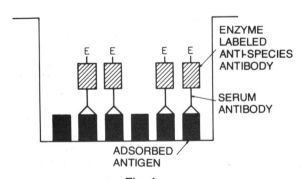

Fig. 1

BINDING SEQUENCE FOR INDIRECT SOLID-PHASE EIAs.

Table I

PREPARATION OF COATING BUFFER (2) FOR ANTIGEN ADSORPTION

Na_2CO_3	1.59 g
$NaHCO_3$	2.93 g
NaN_3	0.20 g
Distilled H_2O	1000 ml

added, where it binds (in the case of a positive serum sample) to the antibody already attached to the antigen. The length of conjugate incubation is also quite variable from assay to assay. Following another wash sequence, substrate is provided for the bound enzyme, which in turn is catalyzed to form a colored reaction product. The test result can be read visually or can be digitized by colorimetric or spectrophotometric means. Because the conjugates are directed toward bound antibody, one conjugate can be used for a variety of etiologic agents which infect a given species. Table II presents an abbreviated list of some of the diseases for

Table II

SELECTED APPLICATIONS OF INDIRECT SOLID-PHASE EIAs FOR THE DETECTION OF ANTIBODY

Antibodies against	Reference
Trichinella spiralis	Ruitenberg et al, 1976 Saunders, 1977
Echinococcus granulosus	Bout et al, 1975
Plasmodium species	
Schistosoma mansoni	Voller et al, 1976
Trypanosoma species	
Brucella abortus	Carlsson et al, 1976; Saunders et al, 1977
Escherichia coli	Jodal et al, 1974
Vibrio cholerae	Holmgren and Svennerholm, 1973
Typhus rickettsiae	Halle et al, 1977
Hog cholera virus	Saunders, 1977; Saunders et al, 1977
Herpes simplex virus	Gilman and Docherty, 1977
Rubella virus	Gravell et al, 1977
DNA (double-stranded)	Standefer et al, 1978

which indirect EIA's have been developed.

B. Double-Antibody Solid-Phase Enzyme Immunoassay

Double-antibody solid-phase EIA's can be used to detect large molecular weight antigens such as bacterial toxins, soluble protein antigens from infectious agents, and viruses. In theory, at least two epitopes must be present per molecule of antigen. In practice, however, the sensitivity of the assay should increase in relation to the number and distribution of epitopes available. The binding sequence of a double-antibody solid-phase EIA is illustrated in Figure 2.

First, antibody (as specific and pure as possible) to the antigen in question is bound to the solid phase, again usually by adsorption techniques but occasionally by covalent linkage (Kato *et al*, 1977; Halpert and Anken, 1977). Suspect material is then incubated with the adsorbed antibody (15 minutes to several hours), and if antigen is present, it will bind to its antibody. Following a wash sequence, antibody conjugated to an enzyme is added to the reaction vessel. If antigen was bound during the prior incubation, the conjugated antibody should bind to the remaining epitopes. After another wash sequence, substrate is provided, and the resulting reaction product is quantitated colorimetrically or spectrophotometrically. Table III lists some of the published applications of double-antibody solid-phase EIA's.

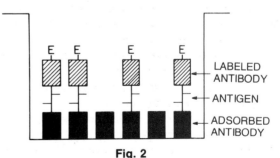

Fig. 2

BINDING SEQUENCE FOR DOUBLE-ANTIBODY SOLID-PHASE EIAs.

Table III

SELECTED APPLICATIONS OF DOUBLE-ANTIBODY SOLID-PHASE EIAs

Antigen detected	Reference
IgG	Kato et al, 1977
Factor VIII	Voller et al, 1976
Alpha-fetoprotein (rat and human)	Maiolini and Masseyeff, 1975
Staphylococcus enterotoxin A	Saunders and Bartlett, 1977
Human chorionic gonadotropin	Van Weemen and Schuurs, 1971
Hepatitis B surface antigen	Wolters et al, 1976
Herpes simplex virus	Mills et al, 1978

C. Competitive Binding Solid-Phase Enzyme Immunoassay

Competitive binding type solid-phase EIA's can be used to quantitate both macromolecular and haptenic substances. For haptens, one must devise a suitable chemical procedure for linking the molecule to the enzyme such that hapten specificity for its antibody is not altered. One must also consider that alteration of the affinity constant for antibody of labeled vs. nonlabeled molecules is possible.

The binding sequence for competitive binding EIA's is illustrated in Figure 3. First, antibody is bound to the surface of the solid phase (e.g., a microplate). Enzyme-labeled antigen is added to one set (one or more) of wells, while enzyme-labeled antigen plus unlabeled "unknown" antigen is added to a second set of wells. After a suitable incubation period, the reaction vessels are washed, and substrate is added to the wells.

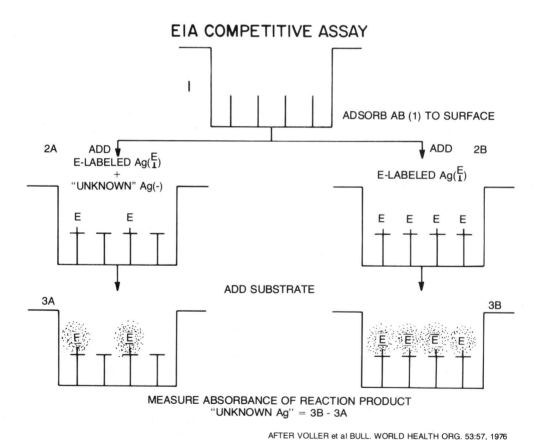

EIA COMPETITIVE ASSAY

MEASURE ABSORBANCE OF REACTION PRODUCT
"UNKNOWN Ag" = 3B - 3A

AFTER VOLLER et al BULL. WORLD HEALTH ORG. 53:57, 1976

Fig. 3

BINDING SEQUENCE FOR COMPETITIVE BINDING EIAs.

Again after a suitable incubation period, the reaction is stopped, and the absorbance of the reaction product present in each well is determined. The amount of unknown antigen present is determined by subtracting the absorbance of the unknown from the absorbance of labeled antigen only and plotting the result against a standard curve. Table IV lists several applications of competitive binding EIA's.

Table IV

SELECTED APPLICATIONS OF COMPETITIVE BINDING EIAs

Antigen detected	Reference
IgG	Engvall and Perlmann, 1971
Alpha-fetoprotein	Belanger et al, 1973
Carcinoembryonic antigen	Engvall and Perlmann, 1975
Human chorionic gonadotropin	Van Weemen and Schuurs, 1971
Insulin	Kato et al, 1976
Thyroid stimulating hormone	Miyai et al, 1976
Cortisol	Ogihara et al, 1977
Gentamicin	Standefer and Saunders, 1978
Aflatoxin B_1	Lawellin et al, 1977

3. Operational Considerations

A. Choice of the Enzyme Amplifier

A list of enzymes used as amplifiers for heterogeneous EIA's is presented in Table V. The most commonly used enzymes have been alkaline phosphatase, β-galactosidase, and horseradish peroxidase (HRP). A single enzyme may not

Table V

ENZYME LABELS USED FOR SOLID-PHASE EIAs

Acetylcholinesterase	Glucoamylase
Alkaline phosphatase	Glucose oxidase
β-D-Galactosidase	Horseradish Peroxidase
Carbonic anhydrase	

be suitable for every EIA performed at any single laboratory. Criteria used in choosing an enzyme amplifier for a particular assay include (1) turnover number (how fast does the enzyme convert substrate?); (2) sensitivity and safety of available substrate systems (certain chromogens used with HRP are carcinogenic, such as diaminobenzidene); (3) ability to couple the enzyme to the desired molecule without greatly altering enzyme activity; (4) stability of the conjugate produced; (5) availability and cost of the enzyme; (6) possible interference of test fluids with the enzyme system (for example, free hemoglobin may nonspecifically bind to the solid phase where it can catalyze substrates used in HRP EIA's); and (7) molecular weight of the conjugates obtained. This becomes especially important if the conjugate must penetrate cell membranes, as in indirect cell-bound virus EIA's [e.g., hog cholera (Saunders, 1977)].

B. Choice of Solid Phase

A variety of materials and configurations have been used as solid phase, some of which are listed in Table VI.

Table VI

SOLID PHASES USED IN EIAs

Cellulose acetate discs

Polystyrene and polyvinyl tubes, discs, beads, and microplates

Glass rods and beads

Tissue culture cells

Sepharose beads

Probably the most commonly used reaction vessel for manual testing is the polystyrene or polyvinyl microtitration tray as it is inexpensive, convenient to use, readily available and, most important, appears to work well for most assays. In the Technicon automated system to be described below, small polystyrene tubes are employed.

C. Binding of Antigen and Antibodies to the Solid Phase

In most assays, binding is accomplished through various adsorptive processes, although covalent linkage has been employed (Kato *et al*, 1977; Halpert and Anken, 1977). The three methods we have used in our work are (1) direct drying of the antigen or antibody to the solid phase (Saunders *et al*, 1977); (2) wet application of antigen or antibody using a special coating buffer (Voller *et al*, 1976); and (3) pretreatment of solid phase with bovine serum albumin (Saunders and Bartlett, 1977). In the first method, one simply dilutes the antigen (or antibody) appropriately and then applies an aliquot (usually 50 to 100μl) to each tube or microplate well, where it is allowed to air-dry. For the second method, the antigen (or antibody) is diluted in the coating buffer (see Table I for composition of the buffer) and aliquoted into the solid phase, which is then sealed to prevent evaporation. Adsorption is allowed to continue for several hours or longer, and the solution can be kept in the reaction vessel until use. In the final method, BSA (200mg/l H_2O) is aliquoted in the amount of 50μl per reaction well or tube, allowed to air-dry, and is then fixed with a 0.25% glutaraldehyde solution for 30 minutes. After thorough washing, 50 to 100μl aliquotes of diluted antigen (or antibody) are added and allowed to air-dry.

The procedure of choice will vary with the assay; it is best, therefore, to try each of these methods for each new assay to determine which one is most efficient. The stability of prepared antigen carriers varies somewhat but usually is on the order of months.

D. Nonspecific Binding: How to Deal With It

Nonspecific binding (NSB) of immunoglobulin, conjugate, or interfering proteins (e.g., hemoglobin in HRP-based assays) to the solid phase can reduce both EIA sensitivity and specificity, especially in those of the indirect type. Binding of these materials to the solid phase is facilitated by aggregation or other denaturation of protein, the presence of large immune complexes and, to some degree, can be related to the relative amounts of protein present in the sample. During incubation periods, all proteins will bind somewhat to available sites remaining on the solid phase. With long incubation periods, all available sites eventually will be occupied by one molecular type or another. Methods to reduce nonspecific binding are designed both to occupy remaining binding sites (after adsorption of either antigen or antibody) and to prevent the firm adsorption of undesired molecules.

The first step of an assay often will include a preliminary incubation step with an indifferent protein such as BSA, or the diluted test fluid may contain BSA in fairly high concentration in relation to potentially interfering proteins. These procedures are designed to bind, preferentially, innocuous molecules to free sites, thus significantly reducing the binding of molecules which can add "noise" to the system. In addition, a nonionic detergent (e.g., Tween 20 or Tween 80) is usually added to incubation fluids as a deterrent to NSB. In our work, we have found that a mildly alkaline, high ionic strength buffer containing Tween 80, when used as a diluting fluid for both serum and conjugate, works very well to prevent significant NSB. The composition of this buffer is 0.5 *M* NaCl, 0.5% Tween 80, and 0.01 *M* PO_4, final pH 8.0.

E. Miscellaneous Considerations

As in all immunoassays, EIA's are dependent on the quality of reagents for their sensitivity and specificity. Where possible, purification procedures should be applied to antigens, antibodies, and conjugates so that precise and accurate results occur with their use. When quantitative assays are performed, it is important also that the reaction product generation follows zero order kinetics. As EIA's often employ microquantities (50 to 100μl) of reagent, deviation from zero order kinetics can occur quite rapidly when significant amounts of enzyme have been bound (due to substrate depletion and/or reaction product inhibition). Finally, methods must be devised to standardize EIA reagents (especially conjugates) such that various laboratories using the same or similar reagents can obtain the same results. More about this important area can be found elsewhere in this volume (Walls, 1979).

4. Automation of Solid-Phase Enzyme Immunoassays

A collaborative effort among the Los Alamos Scientific Laboratory, Technicon Instruments Corporation, and the U.S. Department of Agriculture has resulted in a totally automated processor

for indirect solid-phase EIA's capable of processing up to 300 samples per hour (Saunders *et al*, 1979). With minor modifications, the system can be adapted to sandwich and competitive binding types of EIA's. The configuration of the system is illustrated both photographically (Figure 4) and schematically (Figure 5). Like all Technicon analytical instruments, continuous flow principles are relied on heavily during sample processing. Reference to both Figures 4 and 5 will aid the reader in the following discussion.

Processing rates, incubation times for serum, conjugate and substrate, number of washes, and sample-to-wash ratio are first programmed into the controller at 4 (Figure 5). There are two channels, each of which is processed in the same manner. Cups containing undiluted samples are loaded into the primary sampler at 13, and the sample is picked up and moved through a tube to the proportioning pump at 11, where it is diluted and mixed. The sample then proceeds to the

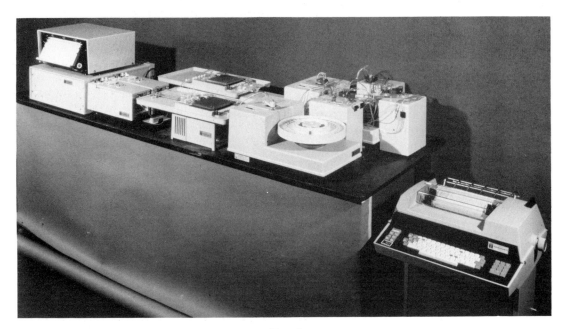

Fig. 4

PHOTOGRAPH OF THE TECHNICON
AUTOMATED EIA PROCESSOR

(Photograph courtesy of Technicon Instruments Corporation, Tarrytown, N.Y.)

TECHNICON EIA RESEARCH SYSTEM

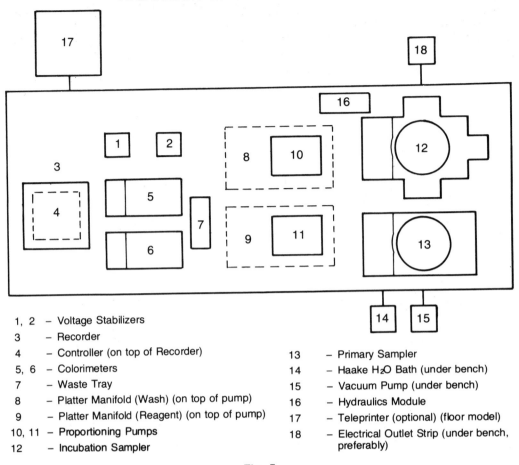

Fig. 5.

SCHEMATIC REPRESENTATION OF THE TECHNICON AUTOMATED EIA PROCESSOR

(Courtesy of Technicon Instruments Corporation, Tarrytown, N.Y.)

1, 2	–	Voltage Stabilizers
3	–	Recorder
4	–	Controller (on top of Recorder)
5, 6	–	Colorimeters
7	–	Waste Tray
8	–	Platter Manifold (Wash) (on top of pump)
9	–	Platter Manifold (Reagent) (on top of pump)
10, 11	–	Proportioning Pumps
12	–	Incubation Sampler
13	–	Primary Sampler
14	–	Haake H₂O Bath (under bench)
15	–	Vacuum Pump (under bench)
16	–	Hydraulics Module
17	–	Teleprinter (optional) (floor model)
18	–	Electrical Outlet Strip (under bench, preferably)

incubation sampler at 12 and is deposited into an antigen-containing tube. Serum incubation, serum wash, conjugate application and incubation, conjugate wash, substrate application and incubation, and reaction product pickup are all performed in the incubation sampler, which contains a temperature-controlled water bath.

After reaction product pickup, the sample is transported through the proportioning pump at 10, where it is diluted before it proceeds through a colorimeter at 5 and 6 and thence to waste. The signal obtained from the colorimeter is transmitted to the recorder at 3, where a graphical readout of each sample occurs. Positive samples are those whose signal in chart divisions is greater than a threshold value determined by running standard negative-control samples. Figure 6 diagrammatically illustrates the sample pathway through the EIA system.

5. Summary

Solid-phase enzyme immunoassays are becoming increasingly popular due to their sensitivity, simplicity, and ver-

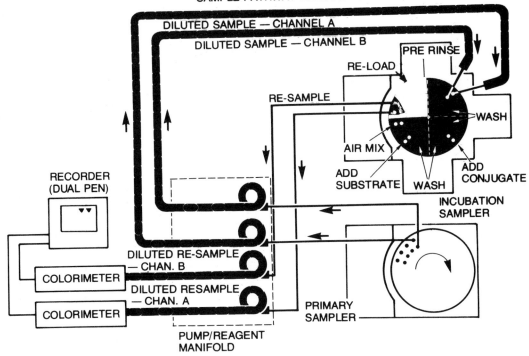

Fig. 6

DIAGRAMMATIC ILLUSTRATION OF THE SAMPLE PATHWAY
THROUGH THE TECHNICON EIA PROCESSOR

(Courtesy of Technicon Instruments Corporation, Tarrytown, N.Y.)

satility. The three most common types of these assays (indirect, double-antibody, and competitive binding) have been described and examples given of their use. Short discussions of various aspects of the "art" of performing solid-phase EIA's have been included. Finally, a brief overview of the Technicon automated EIA processor has been presented.

Acknowledgment

This work was supported by the United States Department of Agriculture (Animal and Plant Health Inspection Services) and the United States Department of Energy under an interagency agreement.

6. References

Belanger, L., Sylvestre, C. and Dufour, D. (1973). *Clin Chim Acta* 48, 15-21

Bout, D., Dugiomont, J. C., Farag, H. and Capron, A. (1975). *Lille Medicale* 20, 561-66

Carlsson, H. E., Hurvell, B., and Linberg, A. A. (1976). *Acta Pathol Microbiol Scand*, Sec. C, 84, 168-76

Engvall, E. and Perlmann, P. (1971). *Immunochem* 8, 871-74

Engvall, E. and Perlmann, P. (1975). *In* "Automation in Microbiology and Immunology" (Heden, T. G. and Illeni, T., eds.), John Wiley & Sons, Inc., New York

Gilman, S. C. and Docherty, J. J. (1977). *J Inf Dis* 136S, S286-94

Gravell, M., Dorsett, P. H., Gutenson, O. and Ley, A. C. (1977). *J Inf Dis* 136S, S300-03

Halle, S., Dasch, G. A. and Weiss, E. (1977). *J Clin Microbiol* 6, 101-10

Halpert, S. P. and Anken, M. (1977). *J Inf Dis* 136S, S318-23

Holmgren, J. and Svennerholm, A. M. (1973). *Infect Immunol* 7, 759-63

Jodal, U., Ahlstedt, S., Carlsson, B., Hanson, L. A., Lindberg, U. and Sohl, A. (1974). *Int Arch Allergy* **47**, 537-46

Kato, K., Hamaguchi, Y., Fukui, H. and Ishikawa, E. (1975). *J Biochem* **78**, 235-37

Kato, K., Hamaguchi, Y., Okawa, S., Ishikawa, E., Kobayashi, K. and Katunuma, N. (1977). *J Biochem* **82**, 261-77

Lawellin, D. W., Grant, D. W. and Joyce, B. K. (1977). *Appl Env Microbiol* **34**, 94-96

Maiolini, R. and Masseyeff, R. (1975). *J Immunol Meth* **8**, 223-39

Mills, K. W., Gerlach, E. H., Bell, J. W., Farkas, M. E. and Taylor, R. J. (1978). *J Clin Microbiol* **7**, 73-76

Miyai, K., Ishibashi, K. and Kumahara, Y. (1976). *Clin Chim Acta* **67**, 263-67

Ogihara, T., Miyai, K., Nishi, K., Ishibashi, K. and Kumahara, Y. (1977). *J Clin End Metab* **44**, 91-95

Ruitenberg, E. J., Steerenberg, P. A., Brosi, B. J. M. and Buys, J. (1976). *J Immunol Meth* **10**, 67-83

Saunders, G. C. (1977). *Am J Vet Res* **38**, 21-25

Saunders, G. C. and Bartlett, M. L. (1977). *Appl Env Microbiol* **34**, 518-22

Saunders, G. C., Campbell, S., Saunders, W. M. and Martinez, A. (1979). *In* "Immunoassays in the Clinical Laboratory" (Nakamura, R. M., ed.) Alan Liss, Inc., New York

Saunders, G. C., Clinard, E. H., Bartlett, M. L. and Sanders, W. M. (1977). *J Inf Dis* **136S**, S258-66

Schuurs, A. H. W. M. and Van Weemen, B. K. (1977). *Clin Chim Acta* **81**, 1-40

Standefer, J. C. and Saunders, G. C. (1978). *Clin Chem* **24**, 1903-07

Standefer, J. C., Saunders, G. C. and Tung, K. S. K. (1978). Submitted for publication

Van Weemen, B. K. and Schuurs, A. H. W. M. (1971). *FEBS Letter* **15**, 232-36

Voller, A., Bartlett, A. and Bidwell, D. E. (1976). *Trans Roy Soc Trop Med Hyg* **70**, 98-106

Voller, A., Bidwell, D. E. and Bartlett, A. (1976). *Bull WHO* **53**, 55-65

Walls, K. (1979). *In* "Diagnostic Immunology: Current and Future Trends" (Keitges, P. W. and Nakamura, R. M., eds.) College of American Pathologists, Skokie, Illinois

Wolters, G., Kuijpers, L., Kacaki, J. and Schuurs, A. (1976). *J Clin Path* **29**, 873-79

CHAPTER III

Future Trends and Application of Immunoassays

P. NAKANE, Ph.D.

Table of Contents

1. Introduction

The use of enzyme labels in immunoassays has progressed rapidly in the past five years. Already several comprehensive reviews of the subject have been published (Wisdom, 1976; Scharpe *et al*, 1976; Dellamonica *et al*, 1977; Schuurs and Van Weemen, 1977) and several international conferences have been held (Leiden, 1974; Paris, 1975; San Diego, 1978; Vienna, 1978). In addition, several developing countries are planning introductory laboratory courses to teach the method. Behind these developments is the realization that the use of enzyme markers gives a rather high level of sensitivity because of the amplifying ability of the enzyme and avoids the difficulties of obtaining and handling radioactive markers. The measurement of enzymatic activity requires no sophisticated and expensive instrumentation as does radioactivity measurement.

In spite of the widespread use of the enzyme immunoassay method, it has not been widely adopted by the clinical laboratories of American institutions for technological reasons. No one has yet been able to develop a fully automated system which can be readily incorporated into the automated systems existing in most clinical laboratories.

Almost all currently available immunoassay systems, regardless of whether they employ enzyme or radioisotope markers, require a step to separate one component from another. If one uses labeled antigen and unlabeled antibody, one must separate antibody-bound antigen from free antigens; similarly, if one uses unlabeled antigen and labeled antibody, one must separate antigen-bound antibody from free antibody. The need for such separation steps has hindered automation (Schuurs and Van Weemen, 1977).

Unfortunately, the majority of techno-logical improvements have been on the separation technique and very little emphasis has been placed on developing a method which avoids a separation step totally. Because of the physical properties of radioisotopes, one cannot avoid the separation step when radioactive tracers are used. On the other hand, enzymes, when used as label, capitalize upon their activity, hence one should be able to manipulate the activity in such a manner that one can distinguish between the activity of enzymes in the presence of immune complexes and in the absence of complexes. Only one method, the EMIT (enzyme-multiplied immunoassay technique) method, has been developed which requires no separation (Rubenstein *et al*, 1972). Although this method has been successfully used to quantitate haptenic antigens, its principle prohibits its use for larger antigens.

However, in the future, nonseparating or homogenous immunoassay methods should be developed rather rapidly. The following will illustrate how this kind of approach may be expanded in three different ways.

2. Modification of the Complement Immunoassay System

When a known amount of complement is reacted with a solution of antigen and a known amount of antibody, some complement will be fixed by antigen-antibody complexes, and the remaining complement can be assayed by its ability to lyse red blood cell (RBC)-anti RBC complexes. The amount of hemoglobin released by the lysed cells can be measured by optical density (at 413nm) and related to the amount of antigen present in the original solution. With this method, one can detect the amount of hemoglobin released from 10^5 RBC's (assuming 0.01 O.D. units to be discriminatable) and can quantitate 1-10ng of antigen (Wasserman and Levine, 1961).

The lysed RBC's also release catalase. Measurement of the released catalase activity should be a much more sensitive assay of lysis than optical density measurement of hemoglobin because of the amplification property of enzyme assays. Our preliminary results, based on spectrophotometric measurement of hydrogen peroxide (H_2O_2) consumption (Beers and Sizer, 1952) indicate that approximately 2×10^{-7} units of catalase are released from each RBC, and thus total hemolysis of 1×10^9 RBC should result in the release of about 200 units of catalase. Unfortunately, we are unable to measure just the released catalase activity in the presence of unlysed RBC; a separation step to remove the unlysed cells is required.

On the other hand, one can sensitively measure hemolysis without separating lysed from unlysed RBC by determining the peroxidase activity of hemoglobin. We have found that the peroxidase activity of hemoglobin cannot be demonstrated in intact unfixed RBC by routine enzyme histochemistry and assume this is due to failure of the hydrogen donor (such as α-naphthol, benzidine, etc.) to penetrate the intact RBC membrane. The H_2O_2 substrate does penetrate, as demonstrated by the catalase activity of intact RBC. We have found the determination of the peroxidase activity of hemoglobin, using a H_2O_2-5-aminosalicylic acid (ASA) method (Van Weemen and Schuurs, 1971), to be a 10-fold more sensitive assay for hemoglobin than optical density measurement. If the spectrofluorometric assay using p-cresol as the hydrogen donor (Roth, 1969) is used, we expect to measure hemoglobin with 100-fold greater sensitivity than is possible by spectrophotometric measurement.

3. Development of a System Requiring Antigen-Antibody Complex Formation for Peroxidase Activity

Both catalase and peroxidase utilize H_2O_2 as substrate. Catalase uses another molecule of H_2O_2 as the hydrogen donor, while peroxidase requires a different hydrogen donor, such as ASA or 4-Cl-1-naphthol (Roth, 1969). Thus, in a solution containing H_2O_2 and ASA, catalase and peroxidase compete for H_2O_2. According to our preliminary results, approximately 180 units of catalase are required per 0.2 unit of peroxidase to cause a 90% reduction in peroxidase activity (in the presence of the H_2O_2 generated by 3.1 units of glucose oxidase).

The H_2O_2 substrate can be generated by various enzymatic systems. For example, the oxidation of glucose by glucose oxidase yields H_2O_2. In a solution containing glucose, glucose oxidase, ASA, peroxidase, and catalase, one would expect the peroxidase and catalase to compete for the H_2O_2 generated by glucose oxidase. If the peroxidase and glucose oxidase are in very close proximity, one would further expect the peroxidase to have an advantage over catalase in the competition for H_2O_2.

Such a close approximation of peroxidase and glucose oxidase should be attainable in an antigen-antibody complex involving two labeled antibodies, one labeled with peroxidase and one labeled with glucose oxidase. In such a system, the peroxidase activity should be proportional to the extent of antigen-antibody complex formation. A similar effect should be achieved by using peroxidase-labeled antigen and glucose oxidase-labeled antibody, or peroxidase-labeled antibody and glucose oxidase-labeled complement 1q (C1q).

4. Development of an Immunoassay System Involving the Reconstitution of Apoperoxidase with Heme and Consequent Restoration of Peroxidase Activity

HRPO contains a heme molecule which is noncovalently bound to the apoperoxidase portion of the enzyme. The heme can be dissociated from the apoperoxidase in acidic media, and the peroxidase activity can be restored by the simple addition of heme (Theorell, 1951; Maehly, 1952). Whether or not heme attached to some other compound, such as an antigen, could also complex with apoperoxidase and thus restore peroxidase activity is unknown. If it can, the principle would offer another possible means for developing an immunoassay system requiring no separation. One such example is as follows:

Microperoxidase (prepared from cytochrome c by pepsin and trypsin digestion) is comprised of an 11 amino acid polypeptide covalently linked through cysteines at the 5th and 8th position to a heme residue (Harburg and Loach, 1960). Microperoxidase may be further digested with pronase to yield heme with two attached cysteine residues. Using the amino terminal of such a cysteine residue or the carboxyl group of heme or cysteine, one may couple the heme to antigen (Means and Feeney, 1971). The heme-antigen conjugate will then be tested for its ability to couple with apoperoxidase and generate peroxidase activity.

If this approach is unsuccessful, a spacer, such as L-lysine or other diamino compounds, may be incorporated between the heme and antigen portions of the conjugate. Perhaps binding of the conjugate to apoperoxidase would be facilitated by enzymatic removal of some of the surface carbohydrate of apoperoxidase. The heme-antigen will then be reacted with antibody and apoperoxidase. One would expect preferential binding of the apoperoxidase to the free heme-antigen rather than to heme-antigen already complexed to antibody. In the presence of unlabeled antigen, the amount of peroxidase activity in the system should be proportional to the amount of unlabeled antigen present.

One other direction where the method may be modified in the near future is that of simplification in processing, such as development of a dip stick. Such developments will bring the method into the offices of the practicing physician; however, at this time, these remain unexplored. Other minor improvements on the conventional enzyme immunoassay will also continue, such as the development of new substrates and soft wares.

Predicting the future of any method is equivocal by nature, and the reader is advised to consult other authors for a more comprehensive understanding of upcoming trends in this area.

5. References

Beers, R. F. and Sizer, I. W. (1952). *J Biol Chem* **195**, 133

Dellamonica, C., Baltassat, P. and Collombel, C. (1977). *Lyon Pharmaceutique* **28**, 289-303

Feder, N. (1970). *J Histochem Cytochem* **18**, 911

Harburg, H. A. and Loach, P. A. (1960). *J Biol Chem* **235**, 364

Leiden (1974). Fifth International Conference on Immunofluorescence and Related Staining Techniques

Maehly, A. C. (1952). *Biochim Biophys Acta* **8**, 1

Means, G. E. and Feeney, R. E. (1971). "Clinical Modification of Proteins," Holden-Day, San Francisco

Paris (1975). First International Symposium on Immunoenzymatic Techniques

Roth, M. (1969). *In* "Methods of Biochemical Analysis" (Glick, D., ed.) p. 236, vol. 17, Interscience, New York

Rubenstein, D., Schneider, E. and Ullman, E. (1972). *Biochem Biophys Res Commun* **47**, 856

San Diego (1978). Immunoassay in the Clinical Laboratory

Scharpe, S. L., Cooreman, W. M., Blomme, W. J. and Laekeman, G. M. (1976). *Clin Chem* **22**, 733

Schuurs, A. H. W. M. and Van Weemen, B. K. (1977). *Clin Chim Acta* **81**, 1

Theorell, H. (1951). *In* "The Enzymes II, Part I," pp. 397-427, Academic Press, New York

Van Weemen, B. K. and Schuurs, A. H. W. M. (1971). *FEBS Letter* **15**, 232

Vienna (1978). Sixth International Conference on Immunofluorescence and Related Staining Techniques

Wasserman, E. and Levine, L. J. (1961). *J Immunol* **87**, 290

Wisdom, G. B. (1976). *Clin Chem* **22**, 1243

CHAPTER **IV**

Quality Control and Standards in Immunoenzyme Assays

K. W. WALLS, Ph.D.

Table of Contents

1. Introduction

Although enzyme immunoassays (EIA) are used for various purposes, this discussion deals only with the application of EIA to antibody detection. Although the procedure was originally designated ELISA (enzyme-linked immunosorbent assay) (Engvall and Perlmann, 1971), it now seems more appropriate to use the general term EIA. To date, no EIA standards have been provided upon which to base quality control. In some cases rather good previous serologic procedures can be used as guidelines, but actual quality control is not yet a functional reality.

Perhaps the first question to ask is what is a standard procedure? To some, this implies a procedure for which each step is explicitly described and must be followed exactly. However, even when well-defined procedures are meticulously performed, exact or reproducible answers are not guaranteed. To others, a standard procedure is simply one which produces the expected end product when tested against a standard.

Clearly, the ultimate goal is to obtain the reproducible correct answer. However, to paraphrase, "no lab is an island"; its personnel must continuously interact with the personnel of other laboratories. Consequently, specimens are submitted to more than one laboratory, reagents are exchanged, and, most importantly, reagent manufacturers must be able to provide satisfactory reagents to all. These factors dictate that a standard procedure be one which is completely and precisely described and performed without deviation in all laboratories. In order to attain such a goal, we must analyze all of the variables of the procedure in question and determine what modifications are needed. Unfortunately for our purpose, some variables such as the marker enzyme are subjectively rather than objectively selected.

2. Solid Substrates

A number of reports describe polystyrene as the most suitable solid substrate. Investigators have used microtitration plates (Voller *et al*, 1974), polystyrene tubes (Ruitenberg *et al*, 1974), latex-coated beads, paper discs (Halbert and Anken, 1977), Sephadex beads (Miranda *et al*, 1977), and polystyrene microcuvettes (Leinikii and Passilla, 1977). All of these have been successfully coated with antigen and used in EIA. We limited our investigation to microtitration plates and evaluated those offered by several manufacturers, including the special MicroELISA plate by Dynatech. We found that the applicability of these products varies with the antigen used. Dynatech (and Greiner Co.) markets a MicroELISA plate which purportedly is superior to all other microtitration plates.

When we used the toxoplasmosis system with horseradish peroxidase and ABTS as the chromogen and compared four microtitration plates [the MicroELISA, Cooke polystyrene (PS), Linbro polystyrene, and the Cooke polyvinyl chloride (PVC)], only minor variations in reactivity occurred. The designs of both the Cooke PS and the Linbro PS are flawed in that these plates have a glare around each well which causes some difficulty in reading. Also, the reactions are perhaps one well lower in these two plates than in the other two tested. The MicroELISA and Cooke PVC elicit comparable reactions, although the reactions in the PVC appear somewhat more intense. With the PVC, although slightly stronger reactions can be obtained, one deals with a flexible plate more difficult to handle. The rigid MicroELISA plate is easier to use but produces slightly weaker reactions and costs nearly three times as much as the PVC. Obviously, neither is the ideal plate.

Either plate can be read visually or with a microcuvette spectrophotometer.

For serodiagnostic purposes, visual readings have proven to be entirely satisfactory. Because of the inherent differences in antigens and the variation in adsorptive qualities of the support matrices, no standard plate can be recommended at this time.

3. Antigens

Antigens can and should be standardized. However, because of the magnitude of such an endeavor, this variable will probably be the last standardized. The antigens for each test must be individually compared and evaluated. One such evaluation to select a standard complement fixation antigen for Chagas' disease took the Pan American Health Organization five years and involved four laboratories before a standard could be established (Alemida, 1972). Because of the international impact, these sorely-needed evaluations should be carried out under the auspices of an international authority after priorities have been established.

4. Washing Methods

Washing represents perhaps one of the biggest and most easily solved problems encountered in the procedure. Simple flooding and shaking the diluent from the plates is inadequate unless extremely carefully done. The size and shape of each well allows droplets of diluent to be trapped and held or air bubbles to form and prevent the well from being filled. By delivering the diluent from a tube with a small orifice, one can direct the stream precisely into each well. Even despite such precautionary measures, air bubbles may form, and the wells may be incompletely washed.

Removing the diluent is even more difficult. Simply inverting and shaking the plate frequently does not affect the contents of some wells. This problem can usually be solved by vigorously rapping the plate on an absorbent towel placed on a flat surface. Of course, if one is working with an infectious antigen or with sera potentially contaminated with hepatitis or other agents, shaking the plates must be avoided. In such a case, one solution is to use a small-tipped suction tube, such as a Pasteur pipette, attached to a side-arm flask. The pipette can be rapidly and easily moved from well to well and the contents aspirated into a disinfectant solution.

Another method uses an instrument (Dynatech Corporation) which sequentially fills and aspirates all 12 wells in a row simultaneously. At each of the 12 positions is a delivery tip and an aspiration tip. Depressing the manifold activates the vacuum, which aspirates the solution into a side-arm flask that may contain disinfectant. Depressing the control lever introduces fresh diluent. The plate is then advanced and the process repeated. It should be noted that this instrument can only be used for washing and aspirating; measured amounts of diluent cannot be introduced. A model which can deliver measured amounts and is more convenient to use was displayed at the 1978 ASM national meeting but has not yet been marketed.

5. Control Sera

Perhaps the most likely standard reagent to be readily available is control serum. Several such products are currently available from WHO, and although few have been evaluated in terms of EIA activity, they have been well-characterized by other procedures and can readily be adapted to enzyme techniques. As is true with antigens, the variety of such products required for all tests makes selecting control sera a gigantic task, although it is probably the least problematic variable of those we are discussing. Standard sera obviously provide the tool against which all other reagents are to be standardized, and as is true with all other standards, sensitivity, specificity, and reactivity must be defined for each serum.

6. Incubation Conditions

Incubation conditions can markedly influence the reaction. The effects of temperature on the time of incubation are notable, with a rate of increase approximating 5% associated with each degree of temperature increase. Most of us work in air-conditioned laboratories and have a choice of a wide range of incubation temperatures; however, because there are many areas in the world where there is no air conditioning and ambient temperatures vary considerably, it seems reasonable to select a temperature practical for all laboratories. Temperatures of 37°C and 42°C have been used; this range exceeds the ambient temperature in most laboratories. An inexpensive water bath or heater will suffice to maintain these working temperatures. Traditionally, 37°C has been most frequently used, but the fact remains that the higher the temperature, the more likely the reagents are to deteriorate.

7. Conjugates

The International Union of Immunological Societies has initiated a program to standardize the enzyme-labeled antiserum. Initially they selected horseradish peroxidase (HRP) as the marker enzyme and began to prepare a standard reagent of well-characterized anti-Fab conjugate. Although alkaline phosphatase was the enzyme initially used by Engvall and Perlmann (1971), most investigators have since chosen HRP. Since that time, it has become considerably less expensive and a highly stable product.

Several considerations were involved in selecting HRP, and the major objection to this enzyme has been the possibility that 5-amino salacylic acid (5-AS), the chromogen used in the substrate, is a carcinogen. Consequently, researchers have sought satisfactory alternatives. A comparison was made of 5-AS, ortho-phenylene-diamine (O-PD), and 2,2'-azino-di-[3-ethyl-benzthiazoline sulfonate (6)] (ABTS). 5-AS, with a deep purple-brown reaction, and ABTS, with a dark green color, are both easy to read visually. Though not as easily read, O-PD is simply prepared, easily terminated, and highly reactive. Because both ABTS and O-PD are highly reactive, the conjugate can be used at approximately 10-fold higher dilution than is possible with 5-AS.

We have found no documented evidence of the carcinogenic or mutagenic properties of these substances. They are not listed as such in the NIOSH (National Institute for Occupational Safety and Health) *Suspected Carcinogens* catalogue, and personal communication with the NIOSH office in Cincinnati, Ohio, revealed no information in their files to indicate that these substances were classified as carcinogenic or mutagenic hazards. It would seem, then, that the chromogen selection is based to a great extent on the individual investigator rather than on the potential hazard.

8. Reading Instruments

Results can vary greatly depending upon the instruments used or the degree of subjectivity involved in evaluating the visual reaction. In the United States, five instruments are marketed which can read the microquantities used in the microtitration test (i.e., usually 0.1 to 0.25ml). The Technicon colorimeter reads quite reproducibly and accurately but can only read about one sample every 30 seconds. In addition, bubbles must not be allowed to enter the flow cell. Another disadvantage of this machine is that the sample is discharged to waste and thus cannot be retested.

The Dynatech ELISA Reader requires that the sample be manually transferred from the microtitration plate to the spectrophotometer and that results be manually recorded. The European version of this instrument has been extensively used (Voller *et al*, 1977) and has been the basis of several research reports.

One advantage of the Gilford Stasar II spectrophotometer is a semi-automatic sampler which transfers the sample from the microtitration tray to the cuvette. In addition, an automatic data recorder is available as an option. Again, bubbles must not be allowed to enter the system because they distort or destroy the reading, and the sample is irretrievable. Of the available instruments, this excellent spectrophotometer seems superior for microdeterminations.

The Finipipette FP-9 spectrophotometer which was recently introduced into the United States uses special micro-cuvettes and appears to have great potential. Nine disposable cuvettes are molded into a single unit in which the reaction occurs. The cuvettes are read on a nine-channel spectrophotometer which plots the results against a standard on a programmable calculator. Although the machine is relatively expensive, its ease of operation, speed of performance, and automatic manipulation of data make it a most promising piece of equipment.

Clem and Yolken (1978) at the National Institutes of Health recently introduced a plate reader which reads directly through the microtitration plate. Although the device is still in the developmental stage, manufacturers have shown interest in modifying and producing it. Totally manually operated, the instrument can be used rapidly and easily, and the sample is retained for any necessary followup testing. Although the plate reader is not as precise and accurate as the spectrophotometers, it provides at least 90% reproducible results, and most of its imprecision is caused by the optical distortion of the plate. For most practical purposes this level of variation is within acceptable limits for serological test results. However, for precise research applications a spectrophotometer should still be used.

9. Techniques for Reporting Results

One of the greatest variables in the procedure is the method of reporting results. Figure 1 illustrates a typical serum titration curve and six methods of reporting the results. Method 1 requires considerable mathematical manipulation,

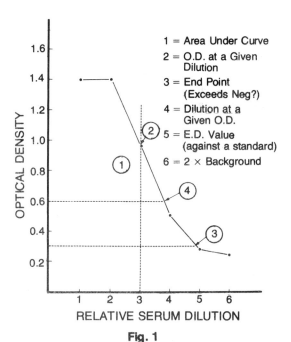

1 = Area Under Curve
2 = O.D. at a Given Dilution
3 = End Point (Exceeds Neg?)
4 = Dilution at a Given O.D.
5 = E.D. Value (against a standard)
6 = 2 × Background

Fig. 1

METHODS FOR DETERMINING SERUM TITERS

but the area under the reaction curve can be determined as an expression of the reactivity of the serum.

Method 2 is one of the most commonly used, and involves determining the optical density at a given dilution and either comparing it to a standard or defining it as a positive when it exceeds a predetermined value. Standardizing this method requires that both parameters be defined: the dilution to be tested and the definition of positive.

Method 3 is only applicable in those systems in which minimal or "0" reactivity is easily identified. The classical definition of the end point is that it is the highest dilution with measurable reactivity. Since some minimal background reactivity occurs in most EIA tests, end points must be described in terms of being equal to the background or not exceeding the negative control. When end points are sharp and background is minimal, this scale is practical and simple to use.

Another of the more common techniques is determining the dilution on the basis of a predetermined optical density (OD). This method is perhaps the most objective of those described, in that it does not depend upon the reactivity of a standard or on a pool of positive or negative sera. When an OD sufficiently above background is used, a quantitative measurement of activity of each specimen can be obtained which is independent of the reactivity level of any other specimen.

The ED or effective dose method is used primarily by Leinikii and Passila (1977) and is a technique borrowed from radioimmunoassay (RIA) methodology. With a programmable calculator, a standard serum curve can be established, and each specimen can be evaluated against it to determine an equivalent value which Leinikii calls the "effective dose." Major questions regarding this procedure are: What are standard sera and standard curves? Do all sera react similarly, or must one select an "average" serum for the standard?

Finally, method 6 is another adaptation of RIA methodology. As was mentioned earlier, many EIA reactions involve a minimal background reaction. Taking this fact into account, a positive is defined as twice (or some other multiple of) the background OD. This definition assumes either that background is the measurement of negatives or that negatives do not exceed twice the reagent control background level. In many antigen-antibody systems, the small reaction which occurs in negative sera must be taken into consideration.

Regardless of the methods used, the similarity of reactivity among specimens and the slopes of reaction are involved; method 1 assumes common slopes which allow for uniform areas; method 2 assumes a slope which will permit one dilution to measure all reactivity levels; method 3 assumes that all sera "taper" to an end point equally; method 4 assumes that all reactions pass through the end point at an equal angle; method 5 assumes that all sera, regardless of strength, have the same slope and thus can be directly compared; and method 6 assumes that serum reactivity is independent of background reaction of any cause.

Figure 2 illustrates four curves plotted with sera tested for toxoplasmosis using HRP and ABTS. Although differences in the slopes of the low-reaction and high-reaction sera are obvious, differences in the slopes for the two strong reactors are not. Figure 3 shows plots of the mathematical slopes determined from three or more sera at each dilution. It can be seen that there is a regularly increasing slope for each titer level. (The dotted line at 1:256 reflects only two sera tested at this level.) These data clearly show that reactivity slopes must be considered if results are to be interpolated as exact end points.

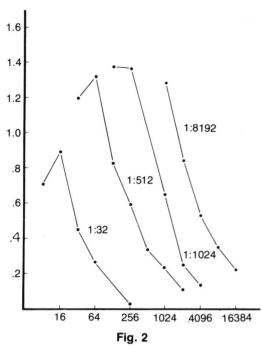

Fig. 2

SERUM SLOPES USING ABTS SUBSTRATE

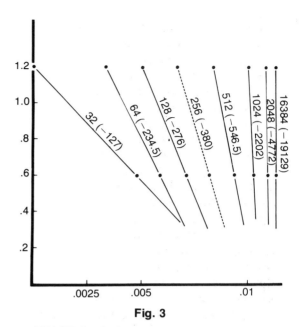

Fig. 3

REACTION SLOPE RELATED TO SERUM
TITER IN ELISA WHEN OPD
IS USED AS SUBSTRATE

10. Conclusion

Quality control and standardization are not yet functional realities in the context of EIA tests. Briefly, we have suggested and illustrated some of the variables which must be evaluated: the solid-phase matrix upon which the reaction is performed; the type and form of antigen adsorbed to the surface; the method of washing and removing reagents from the test; the variabilities involved in the sera being tested; the incubation conditions; the type of conjugate to be prepared with what enzyme; the effects and advantages of various substrates and chromogens; the methods of reading results; and finally, the methods of reporting the results. To date, progress in this endeavor is represented only by the availability of a few international sera and a program recently initiated to prepare a standard conjugate. Clearly, there is much work to be done. With the rapid acceptance of EIA, more effort must be placed on preparing standard reagents and on formulating a unified standard procedure. No method can be successful until reagents are commercially available. Conversely, reagent manufacturers cannot invest in EIA until they are assured of what EIA needs. Standardization can solve both problems, and with standardization will come quality control.

11. References

Alemida, J. O. de. (1972). *In* "Research in Immunochemistry and Immunobiology 2" (Kwapinski, J. B. G., ed.) pp. 247-95, University Park Press, Baltimore

Clem, T. R. and Yolken, R. H. (1978). *J Clin Micro* **7**, 55-58

Engvall, E. and Perlmann, P. (1971). *Immunochem* **8**, 871-74

Halbert, S. P. and Anken, M. (1977). *J Inf Dis* **136S**, 318-23

Leinikii, P. O. and Passila, S. (1977). *J Inf Dis* **136S**, 294-99

Miranda, Q. R., Bailey, G. D., Fraser, A. S. and Tenoso, H. J. (1977). *J Inf Dis* **136S**, 304-17

Ruitenberg, E. J., Steerenberg, P. A., Brosi, B. J. M. and Buys, J. (1974). *Bull WHO* **51**, 108-09

Voller, A., Bidwell, D. E., Bartlett, A. and Edwards, R. (1977). *Trans Roy Soc Trop Med Hyg* **71**, 431-37

Voller, A., Bidwell, D. E., Huldt, G. and Engvall, E. (1974). *Bull WHO* **51**, 209-21

PART 3

DIAGNOSTIC IMMUNOLOGY

CHAPTER **I**

State of the Art of Immunofluorescence Techniques in Tissues*

E. H. BEUTNER, Ph.D., W. L. BINDER, Ph.D., V. KUMAR, Ph.D.

Table of Contents

---

*This research is supported in part by a grant from the Summerhill Foundation.

1. Introduction

Most clinical laboratory work and research on immunofluorescence (IF) of tissue is performed with antibodies to immunoglobulins or complement components labeled with FITC (fluorescein isothiocyanate) [Beutner *et al*, 1968; Beutner and Nisengard, 1973; Goldman, 1968]. These conjugates serve for indirect and direct IF tests. To determine the significance of findings obtained with these (or any other) IF test systems, each of the critical factors and reagents must be controlled and defined reproducibly. For indirect IF tests the following factors are critical:

1. Reference sera specificity and sensitivity
2. Antigenic substrates
3. Conjugate specificity and sensitivity
4. Test conditions and optical system

Reference sera serve as the only required reference standard[1]. The other three factors are defined objectively to render test systems reproducible. This review of the state of the art provides some relevant details on how to achieve reproducibility. Attention to these details (plus some experience) yields results of the type summarized in Table I.

Both of the field trials listed in Table I show that most or all laboratories with trained personnel can achieve titers by indirect IF tests which are reproducible within the tolerance limits of two doubling dilutions (±1 dilution). Both employed selected conjugates; without this, the variation is somewhat greater. Both entailed the use of a single selected tissue antigen; without this, it is impossible to obtain reproducible results. Both were performed by trained personnel with experienced supervisors; without this, IF tests (like any other test) may be expected to yield erratic results. In effect, IF tests are reproducible if performed correctly under defined conditions.

While antinuclear antibodies serve as the primary model for indirect IF test systems in this review, comparable methods can be employed for any other indirect IF test system and have been applied to several [(Beutner *et al*, 1968; Beutner and Nisengard, 1973) See Table IB]. For direct IF studies, particularly of pathologic tissues, we have, in principle, the choice between using objectively defined conjugates which yield reproducible results under standard test conditions and selecting reagents which give "the best" or "the desired" or "typical" staining patterns. The latter is necessary for histologic staining methods and is unfortunately applied in many histochemical studies, but it is clearly contraindicated for reliable immunopathologic studies. Immunochemical assays for evaluating conjugates used for indirect IF studies also afford a functional, and apparently a reliable, basis for selecting reagents for direct IF studies.

2. Reference Sera and Tissue Antigens for Indirect IF Tests

Clinical laboratory tests performed by indirect IF methods are used most commonly for the detection of tissue autoantibodies such as antinuclear antibodies (ANA), antimitochondrial antibodies (AMA), and anti-smooth muscle antibodies (ASMA). They are also used, to some extent, for the detection of antibodies to native DNA as well as to selected infectious agents, e.g. the fluorescent treponemal antibody absorption test and tests for antibodies to *Toxoplasma gondii* and CMV. Reference sera for ANA are available, to a limited ex-

---

[1]As in other test systems, working standards which have been compared to the reference standards serve as controls for routine tests. These two types of standards are distinct from the assay standards used in fluorescein and protein assays.

Table I

REPRODUCIBILITY OF INDIRECT IF TESTS AS REVEALED BY TWO FIELD TRIALS

A. Titers obtained with one antinuclear antibody containing serum (IUIS-WHO reference serum 66/233) in 28 chessboard titrations performed by five laboratories with six commercially prepared conjugates*

conjugate no.:	1	2	3	4	5	6
Laboratory A	100 (150)	400	200 (75)	200 (250)	(300) 200-400 (150)	(300) 200-400 (350)
" B	100-200	100 (240)	50-100	200-300	100-200 (240)	300-400 (240)
" C	160	160-320	160	320	160-320 (120)	160-320 (120)
" D	160	160	160 (240)	160	80-160	80-160
" E	160	160	160-320	NT	NT	320
Variation range:	1.6x	4x	2.7x	2x	2.5x	2.9x
acceptable	x		x	x	x	x
not acceptable		x				

B. Titers obtained with two sera with pemphigus antibodies (PA) and one serum with bullous pemphigoid antibodies (BPA) in 9 laboratories using monkey sections and selected conjugates.

serum no:	PA-1	PA-2	BPA
Laboratory A	640	40	640
B	320	40	640
C	640	40	1280
D	640	80	640
E	320	80	640
F	320	20	320
G	640	80	NT
H	640	(160)**	(2560)**
I	640	40	640
Variation range:	2x	8x**	16x**
acceptable	x		
not acceptable		x	x

*Adapted from data reported in Ann. N.Y. Acad. Sci. *177*, 361, 1971 (ref. 4).
**These are not acceptable titers or titer ranges. The remaining laboratories reported titers in the 4-fold variation range which is acceptable for IF work

tent, through the IUIS-WHO[2] and through the International Service for Immunology Laboratories[3]. The ISIL also supplies undiluted reference sera for comparative studies of AMA, ASMA, pemphigus and pemphigoid antibodies, and antibodies to thyroid cells on a limited basis. Small samples of diluted reference sera are supplied (at very high prices) with commercial kits for ANA, AMA, SMA and DNA antibodies, but these are of little value for comparative studies.

In principle, the specificity of reference sera for tissue autoantibodies should be defined in terms of their immunoglobulin class, species, organs and/or tissues which contain reactive antigens, their titer(s) on selected organs

[2]Dr. Astrid Fagraeus, Department of Immunology, National Bacteriological Laboratory, S 105 21 Stockholm, Sweden (IUIS-WHO)

[3]ISIL is a private non-profit foundation. The supervisor is Dr. Vijay Kumar, 219 Sherman Hall, SUNY/Buffalo, Buffalo, N.Y. 14214

and/or tissues, the patterns of staining where relevant, and the methods of handling the tissues. The latter should include at least the time and temperature of storage, thickness of sections, and any methods of fixation.

In practice, reference sera with ANA of known immunoglobulin classes are difficult to obtain; at present, a limited amount of an ANA of the IgM class (a Wallentröm serum) is available through the IUIS-WHO, and small amounts of an IgG fraction of ANA-containing serum is available through the ISIL. The latter group can also provide pemphigus antibodies of the IgG class. Necessary information on test conditions and titers with the recommended tissue antigens is, for the most part, available through these agencies.

3. Chessboard Titrations

Two-dimensional or chessboard titrations afford the basis for defining indirect IF test systems (Beutner et al, 1968; Beutner, 1971a). They entail tests of serial dilutions of the unlabeled tissue antibodies with serial dilutions of conjugate with known concentrations of antibodies. With the aid of the above-described IgG and IgM class specific ANA, it is possible to test the specificity of commercially-available Ig class specific conjugates. The results of such a study are shown in Table II.

The two-dimensional, or chessboard, titrations of the two reference ANA preparations shown in Table II serve to verify both their Ig class specificity and the class specificity of the anti-Ig antibodies in the first two conjugates used to detect them. This type of system affords the most reliable specificity test for indirect IF studies of Ig class specific reagents from both the qualitative and quantitative standpoint. In the example given in Table II the "plateau titer" of the IgG class ANA was 320 with the

monospecific reagent and 160 to 320 with the polyvalent conjugate. The plateau titer of the IgM class ANA was 160 with both the monospecific and the polyvalent conjugates. These are the ANA titer ranges we may expect with these sera in standard one dimensional titration if an appropriately defined indirect IF test system is used.

4. Critical Factors in the Definition of an Indirect IF Test for ANA

A number of factors, many of which are not detailed in the literature, are of critical importance for indirect IF tests of the type reviewed in Table II. These include the following:

A. Rat liver is frozen in liquid N_2 (other methods are less suitable for 2μ sections) and stored at $-70°C$ for not more than one month. Sections can be stored at $-70°C$ without protection for about one week, but not in solid CO_2. (These factors vary for each tissue antigen.) Sections must be cut at 2μ. Those cut at 4μ or more give sensitivities of ANA tests that are markedly decreased. Also, a poor quality of section may give a weak or negative reaction. If frozen sections are used, they must be air dried for 30 minutes to prevent washing off. They should not be re-frozen.

B. Readings can be made with substage illumination using either UV or BV type filters (Kawamura et al, 1973; Goldman, 1968) or with epillumination using any one of a variety of acceptable filters. While the intensity of illumination may vary by a factor of 10-fold or more, the actual differences in titers observed visually rarely vary by more than one, or at most two, doubling dilutions. This holds true for at least three different light sources (Hg vapor, Xenon, quartz halogen) for epi- or substage

Table II

CHESSBOARD TITRATIONS OF IgG AND IgM CLASS ANA WITH THREE TYPES OF CONJUGATES

Anti-IgG Conjugate (Meloy; see Table III)

		Use Dil.*		Plateau endpoint (PEP)		Plateau titer (PT)			
IgG ANA	640	w+	w+/±	w+/±	±	—			
	320	+	+	+/w+	w+/±	—			
	160	++	+/w+	+/w+	+/w+	—			
	80	+++	++	++	+/w+	—			
	40	+++	++	++	+/w+	—			
NHS*	1/20	—	—	—	—	—			
	1/10	—	—	—	—	—			
IgM ANA	320	—	—	—	—	—			
	160	—	—	—	—	—			
	80	—	—	—	—	—			
	40	—	—	—	—	—			
	1/20	—	—	—	—	—			
NHS	1/10	—	(1/2)	(1/4)	(1/8)	—			
	1/10	—	—	—	—	—			
U/ml* anti-IgG		1/4	(1/2)	1/8	(1/4)		(1/2)	(1/8)	
μg/ml anti-IgG		56	28	14					
U/ml anti-IgM		—	—	—					
Dilution		1/8	1/16	1/16	1/32	1/64	1/8	1/16	1/32 / 1/128

Anti-IgM Conjugate (Meloy; see Table III)

IgG ANA	640	—	—	—	—	—	
	320	—	—	—	—	—	
	160	—	—	—	—	—	
	80	—	—	—	—	—	
	40	—	—	—	—	—	
NHS	1/20	—	—	—	—	—	
	1/10	—	—	—	—	—	
IgM ANA	320	w+	w+	w+/±	w+	—	
	160	+/++	+	+/w+	+	w+	
	80	++	+/w+	++	+/w+	+/w+	
	40	++/+++	++	+++	++	+/++	
	1/20	++/+++	+++	+++	+	+	
NHS	1/10	—	—	—	—	—	
	1/10	—	—	—	—	—	
U/ml anti-IgG		(1)					
U/ml anti-IgM		1/4	(1/2)	1/8	1/16	1/32	1/64
μg/ml anti-IgM		56	28	14	30	15	7	4
Dilution		1/8	1/16	1/16	1/32	1/128	1/256 / 1/512

Anti-Ig Conjugates (polyvalent C458; see Table III)

IgG ANA	640	—	w	±/w	—	+/w	w+	+/w
	320	w	w	w	±/w	+	w+	—
	160	w	+	+	+/++	+/++	++	w+
	80	+/++	+/w	+/w	++/+++	++	+/++	+/w+
	40	++	+/++	++	+++	+++	+++	+
NHS	1/20	+++	+++	w	±/	±	—	—
	1/10	—	—	±/w	—	NSS*	—	—
IgM ANA	320	—	±/w	+/w	+/w	(8)	(4)	(1/4)	(1/8)
	160	—	+	+	+	1	1/2	1/32	1/64
	80	±/w	+	w	w	1/2	1/4	1/64	1/128
	40	+/w	+/++	+/w	+/w			1/64	1/256
NHS	1/10	w	+	±	w/±				
	1/10	±/w	w	±/w	w/±				
U/ml anti-IgG		1/2	(1/16)	1/4	(1/32)	(8)	(4)	(1/8)	(1/16)
U/ml anti-IgM		(1/16)	1/32	1/32	1/64	1	1/2	1/64	1/128
Dilution		1/32	1/64	1/128	1/256	1/512	1/1024	1/128	1/256

*Use dil. = use dilution; NHS = normal human serum; U/ml = units/ml (see text); NSS = nonspecific staining.

illumination and with various acceptable filter combinations. This appears to be due to compensation by the human eye for differences in intensity. Most readings of ANA are made with BV (Goldman, 1968) illumination. The optical system selected must be described in detail and evaluated with reference sera of known titers and conjugates.

C. Conjugate characteristics govern titers by their optical sensitivity ratio (F/P ratio) over a range of about two doubling dilutions. Thus, this factor can be used to compensate for differences in the optical system (point B above).

D. Standard test conditions need to be used (Goldman, 1968). For the tests summarized in Table II the following factors were controlled:

1) time of incubation (30 min. incubation for sera and conjugate),
2) time of second washing after conjugate (at least 10 min. or more),
3) moisture control (even slight desiccation can convert a positive ANA to a negative),
4) purity of H_2O (glass distilled H_2O is best for preparing PBS (phosphate buffered saline) [Beutner, 1971a] for dilution of sera and conjugates, but it is not needed for washing),
5) 10% PBS, 90% glycerol mounting medium (pH 7.2 PBS is used here with a nonfluorescent glycerol), and
6) conjugates of the desired specificities and sensitivities.

5. Conjugate Characterization and Selection

Conjugates must be selected and used on the basis of their relevant characteristics; three basic characteristics of anti-Ig or C or any other conjugates enter into their selection, i.e. their specificity, their optical sensitivity or F/P ratios, and their antibody content. From these and other characteristic multiple deductions, inferences and predictions can be made as indicated in Table III. (The derivation and uses of values listed in Table III are reviewed in the subsections below.) The use of reference conjugates[4] is contraindicated.

Most commercially prepared conjugates marketed in the U.S. by leading manufacturers supply the relevant data needed to characterize them. Since the antibody content decreases on storage, it is advisable to check this. Also, performance tests, preferably in the form of chessboard titration, should be carried out. Dilutions should be expressed on the basis of the antibody content of the conjugate.

A. Data Commonly Supplied by Conjugate Manufacturers

Data supplied by, or derived from, the data supplied by manufacturers are listed in Table III in points 1, 2a to d, 3b and d, and 4. These data, which are provided by most leading conjugate manufacturers, are of value and should be recorded and used.

The data on specificity of reagents are generally reliable as illustrated by the specificity of the anti-IgG and anti-IgM conjugates in the chessboard titrations shown in Table II. Another method for checking the specificity of conjugates in performance tests that we may look to in the future is that of inert beads coated with known amounts of purified Ig or C components.

The data on fluorescein (F) and protein (P) assay values supplied by manufacturers, as well as the F/P ratios calculated from them, are of variable reliability; assays based on 495nm/280nm extinction ratios, which are widely used in Europe (e.g. Burroughs-Wellcome), are not as reliable as F assays run with reference standards (McKinney et al,

---

[4]The IUIS-WHO make two reagents available. As indicated in the section on "reference conjugates" below, these afford no advantages over conjugates that are commercially available. The prime focus of attention should be on the *methods of characterizing* such man-made reagents.

1964) and P assays performed by the biuret method (Beutner, 1971a). The latter two methods are recommended by the NCCLS (Anonymous, 1975) and are employed by most of the leading conjugate manufacturers in the United States.

Carefully controlled studies show that titers of antibodies by indirect IF tests are proportional to the F/P ratios of conjugates (Beutner *et al*, 1968; Shu *et al*,

1975). For example, the molar F/P ratios given in the package inserts of the two monospecific Meloy[5] conjugates fall into the same range as the polyvalent conjugate prepared in this laboratory, as indicated in Table III (2.9 and 3.0 versus

---

[5]Meloy Laboratories, Inc., 6715 Electronic Drive, Springfield, Virginia 22151

Table III
SUMMARY OF DATA ON CONJUGATES AND ON CHESSBOARD TITRATIONS

	Conjugates used for titrations listed in Table II		
1) *Specificity* Lot No.	**anti-IgG** **(Meloy** **77729)**	**anti-IgM** **(Meloy** **77633)**	**anti-Ig** **polyvalent** **(SUNY C458)**
2) *Assays for optical sensitivity (F/P) ratios*			
a) fluorescein	32.2	36.0	69.0
b) protein	11.1	12.0	12.7
c) weight F/P ratio	2.9	3.0	5.4
d) molar F/P ratio	1.2	1.2	2.1
3) *Antibody (Ab) concentration*			
a) anti-IgG U/ml*	4-8**	<1 (neg)	16**
b) " " μg Ab/ml	0.9	neg	ND*
c) anti-IgM U/ml	<1 (neg)	4-8**	2**
d) " " μ Ab/ml	neg	1.9	ND
e) Ratio of μg Ab/U	0.1 to 0.2 μg/U	0.2 to 0.5 μg/U	ND
4) *Less commonly used activity ratios*			
a) molar Ab/P ratio	0.9/11.1 = 0.08	1.9/12 = 0.16	ND
b) molar Ab/F ratio	0.08/1.2 = .067	0.16/1.2 = 0.13	ND
5) *Plateau titers of ANA from Table II*			
a) IgG class ANA	320	<20 (neg)	160-320
b) IgM class ANA	<20 (neg)	160	160
6) *Plateau endpoints (PEP) of conjugate from Table II*			
a) PEP dil.* for IgG-ANA	1/32	NR*	1/256
b) " U/ml " " "	1/4-1/8	"	1/16
c) " μg Ab/ml " "	28	"	ND
d) PEP dil. for IgM-ANA	NR	1/256	1/128
e) " U/ml " " "	"	1/32-1/64	1/64
f) " μg Ab/ml " "	"	7.4	ND
7) *Use dilution of conjugates*			
a) for IgG-ANA (Table II)	1/2 to 1/4 U/ml	NR	1/8 U/ml
b) " " " "	or 56 μg/ml	"	ND
c) for IgM-ANA (Table II)	NR	1/16 to 1/32 U/ml***	1/32 U/ml***
d) " " " "	"	or 15 μg/ml***	ND

e) for all indirect IF
      tests (based on over
      200 chessboard titrations)
	1/4 U/ml or
	 50 μg Ab/ml
		1/4 to 1/8 U/ml or
		 25-50 μg Ab/ml
			1/4 U/ml or
			 50 μg Ab/ml

*ND = not done; NR = no reaction observed; U/ml = units/ml (see text); PEP dil. = plateau endpoint dilution.

**These unitage assays were performed with purified IgG or IgM preparations rather than with normal human sera as suggested in the text. Details of these studies will be reported at a later date by Binder *et al*.

***These values are maximal use dilutions based on the data in Table II. Lower use dilutions can be used and are safer based on past experience. Concentrations should not be over 1/2 U/ml or 100 μg Ab/ml since they tend to give weaker reactions in some IF systems.

NOTE: Subsequent lots of anti-IgM conjugate from Meloy have failed to give comparable reactivity in unitage assays and in IF tests.

2.1). As may be expected, the plateau titers are also comparable for both the IgG and IgM class ANA. In the same series of studies two polyvalent conjugates with lower molar F/P ratios (1.1 and 1.2) yield a lower IgG class ANA titer (i.e. 80). It is a rule of thumb that titers are proportional to F/P ratios if titrations and F and P assays are done correctly.

For IF studies of tissues, molar F/P ratios in the range of 1 to 4.5 are most useful. This affords about a two doubling dilution range in titers that can be obtained with a given serum. As indicated in a preceding section, this range of variation can be used to compensate for variations in the sensitivity of optical systems in obtaining titers with reference sera (such as those described above) that fall into the expected range (see Table I).

The other activity ratios derived from the data provided include the Ab/P and the Ab/F ratio. The two Ab/P ratios of 0.08 and 0.16 listed in Table III indicate that the protein in the anti-IgG and anti-IgM conjugates contain, respectively, 8% and 16% antibody. Polyvalent anti-Ig conjugates should contain 10% or more antibody according to an international agreement (Beutner, 1971b); monospecific reagents sometimes contain less. The Ab/F ratio is proportional to the ratio between the titer of desired specific staining (a function of mg Ab/ml) and the nonspecific staining titer (a function of μg F/ml) of a conjugate for a given set of conditions (Beutner, 1971b). It is not widely used, however.

The antibody protein assays provided by manufacturers can be used as a basis for diluting conjugates as indicated below.

B. Unitage Assays as a Basis for Conjugate Characterization

One crude but functional method of checking on the antibody content of conjugates is the unitage assay. It entails: 1) a simple gel diffusion test, 2) the use of data supplied by manufacturers as described above, and 3) chessboard titrations of the type shown in Table II.

Unitage assays are performed with a central well with 1mg/ml of antigen and six peripheral wells with serial dilutions of conjugate, using a standard template or a linear array of wells containing antigen and conjugated antibodies. The titer or unitage affords a crude, but useful, measure of antibody content, and therefore, also of the dilution for routine titrations of tissue antibodies. Purified Ig preparations are needed for class specific unitage assays. For crude assays, pooled fresh normal serum can be diluted to obtain the desired 1mg/ml concentration of the given Ig class or complement component by using values of their concentration in normal sera. Thus, for example, a 1/12 dilution of pooled normal serum provides about 1mg IgG/ml; a 1/3 dilution gives about 1mg IgA/ml, and undiluted serum can be used for IgM and C3 assays.

One problem with this assay method is that the endpoint readings differ from one laboratory worker to the next (more so than readings of IF titrations). Thus, for example in Table III, points 3a and 3c give ranges of unitage assay readings by two investigators. However, once a worker has established the relationship between the plateau endpoints, or PEP, of conjugates (their highest dilution which still gives a plateau titer) and their unitages as seen in his own laboratory in multiple chessboard titrations, then the unitage alone can be used to select use dilutions for routine tests. The latter should be one to three dilutions before the PEP. Despite the variations in readings of unitages over 240, published chessboard titrations with data on labeled antibody concentrations show that about 90% of PEP fall in the range of 1/8 to 1/32 unit/ml (Beutner *et al*, 1975). As indicated in Table III (points 5 and 6), while the PEP ranged from 1/4 to 1/64 units, and thus apparent use dilutions might range from 1/2 to 1/16 unit/ml, the experience in this laboratory indicates that use dilutions should be adjusted to a narrower range of 1/4 to 1/8 unit/ml.

C. Antibody Protein Assays as a Basis for Conjugate Characterization

Several methods can be used to assay antibody protein of precipitating antibodies of the type used for preparing the anti-Ig and anti-C conjugates for tissue IF studies. A relatively simple one, which requires minimal equipment and which we have found to be useful in IF studies, is a reverse radial immunodiffusion assay (Beutner and Nisengard, 1973; Beutner, 1971a; Beutner, 1971b; Beutner *et al*, 1975). These assays are based on the diameter or area of precipitation rings around wells filled with the antibody containing conjugate in agar plus known antigen concentrations. The reproducibility is in the fair to good range (15% to 40% maximum variation between five laboratories in assays of six conjugates). It is much better than unitage assays.

The readings are less subjective with values in mg Ab/ml rather than titers or units/ml. For example, the PEP values expressed as mg Ab/ml in Tables II and III varied by a factor of fourfold, while the values listed as unitages varied by 16-fold. This represents almost the total range of variation observed in over 240 chessboard titrations (Beutner *et al*, 1975). On the average, one unit is roughly equivalent to 0.2mg Ab/ml (Beutner, 1971a); this is borne out by the data in Table III (point 3e). Thus, the prime value of assays of mg Ab/ml is that they afford a reliable basis for selecting conjugate dilutions for standard one-dimensional titrations of sera. As indicated in Table III (point 7e), a standard dilution recommended for all indirect IF tests is $50\mu g$ Ab/ml of conjugate. The use of concentrations over $100\mu g$ Ab/ml may give less specific staining and more nonspecific than lower concentrations. Assays of mg Ab/ml also permit calculations of Ab/P and Ab/F ratios. These are primarily of value in preparing and/or selecting conjugates, while not as valuable in performance tests.

One problem with reverse radial immunodiffusion assays is that they require reference standards with known antibody content. This can, to some extent, be circumvented by using standard antigen concentrations in the agar and standard curves or by using the assay values supplied by the manufacturer. The former is subject to errors in antigen concentrations in the agar, and the latter is risky because conjugates sometimes lose their antibody activity more rapidly than expected, possibly due to storage at room temperature during shipment.

6. Reference Conjugates

Two reference conjugates are available through the IUIS-WHO, notably in anti-Ig (polyvalent) and an anti-IgM specific reagent. These are characterized by the same methods which are used for assays of the reagents prepared by some of the European manufacturers of conjugates. Ratios of extinctions at 495/280 are given instead of data on F and P content; i.e. F and P assays are not done by the methods recommended by the NCCLS (Anonymous, 1975). They are not as reliable as the NCCLS recommended assays used by most U.S. manufacturers.

As reference reagents these conjugates can, from a practical point of view, be compared with reference reagents and methods now used by industry for assays of these and other conjugates. For assays of FITC and protein concentrations of conjugates, the "reference conjugates" are not, as indicated above, reliable reference reagents. In assays for antibody content they, like commercial conjugates, can serve only as secondary standards. For primary assays of antibody content, these or any other anti-Ig conjugates must be tested, e.g. with immunoabsorbents or with soluble antigens at optimal proportions, for determinations of their content of total mg Ab/ml. In tests for Ig class specificity, the most reliable and relevant assays are performed, as shown in Table II, with antibodies of a single Ig class. Appropriate reference sera serve equally well in the evaluation of the Ig class specificity of the IUIS-WHO reference conjugates as any other conjugates, be they of commercial origin or "home-made." Conversely the "reference conjugates" and any other conjugates which are Ig class specific can serve equally well as reference reagents for identifying the Ig class(es) in tissue or serum antibodies. Tests of sensitivity of conjugates in performance tests with tissue antibodies also rest on the reference sera, as shown in Table II, regardless of the source of the conjugate. Also, regardless of its source, the sensitivity of a conjugate is a function of its F/P ratio and its antibody content.

In brief, while the reference *sera*, e.g. from the IUIS-WHO or ISIL, are of considerable value for achieving reproducibly defined IF test systems, the IUIS-WHO reference *conjugates* do not differ significantly from commercially-prepared conjugates. It seems inappropriate for the IUIS-WHO to go into competition with industry.

Comparative study of the *reliability of objective methods for conjugate assays* and their relevance to reactivity in performance test is a more fruitful endeavor in the definition of and, if desired, the standardization of IF staining procedures than is the preparation of "reference conjugates."

7. Summary: Uses of Reproducibly Defined IF Techniques in Studies of Tissue

With reproducible indirect IF tests it is possible to determine the clinical significance of titers. For example, under the conditions used for the ANA titration shown in Tables IA and II, titers of 40 or more occur in 18% (19/107) of normal control subjects (age 18 to 66, 1/2 male, 1/2 female), titers of 80 or more occur in 6% of normal population, and titers of 160 in only 0.9% (1/107) (Shu et al, 1975). Under the same conditions 89% (23/26) of sera from active cases of SLE had ANA titers of 40 or more, and 85% (22/26) of these cases had ANA titers of 160 (Nisengard et al, 1975). Thus, in screening for ANA with this particular test system, titers of 40 or 80 are of doubtful significance, while titers of 160 are of clinical significance, and titers of 320 or more are highly suggestive of an immunologic disturbance.

The above data on ANA and on pemphigus antibody titers serve merely as examples of the value of reproducible indirect IF titers. Without the use of reproducible IF methods such analyses would not be possible.

The detection of pemphigus antibodies serves not only as a valuable diagnostic aid, but their titers parallel the severity or extent of the bullous eruptions (Beutner et al, 1973). A rise in titer of these antibodies frequently precedes the development of an increase in the severity of the disease, while a drop in titer is a sign of clearing. Thus, titers of pemphigus antibodies can, if determined under properly controlled conditions, serve as an adjunct in the adjustment of dosages of corticosteroid and/or immunosuppressive agents used in the treatment of the disease. Considering the fact that these agents must frequently be used at such high doses that the treatment itself is now a primary cause of death in severe cases of pemphigus, the determination of pemphigus antibody titer, fluctuating under reproducibly defined conditions, assumes obvious importance.

8. References

Anonymous. (1975). "Approved Standard: ASM-1. Standard Test for Labeling Efficiency of Fluorescein Isothiocyanate (FITC)," pp. 1-4, National Committee for Clinical Laboratory Standards, Villanova, Pennsylvania

Beutner, E. H. (1971a). *Ann New York Acad Sci* **177**, 361-403

Beutner, E. H. (1971b). *Ann New York Acad Sci* **177**, 506-26

Beutner, E. H., Chorzelski, T. P., Bean, S. F. and Jordon, R. E., eds. (1973). "Immunopathology of the Skin: Labeled Antibody Studies," 1st ed., Dowden, Hutchinson and Ross, Stroudsburg, Pennsylvania

Beutner, E. H., Deng, J-S, Shu, S., Andersen, P. and Peetoom, F. (1975). *Ann New York Acad Sci* **254**, 573-91

Beutner, E. H. and Nisengard, R. J. (1973). *In* "Immunopathology of the Skin: Labeled Antibody Studies," 1st ed. (Beutner, E. H., Chorzelski, T. P., Bean, S. F. and Jordon, R. E., eds.) Dowden, Hutchinson and Ross, Stroudsburg, Pennsylvania

Beutner, E. H., Sepulveda, M. R. and Barnett, E. V. (1968). *Bull WHO* **39**, 587-606

Goldman, M. (1968). *In* "Fluorescent Antibody Methods," pp. 97-117 and 41-59, Academic Press, New York

Kawamura, A., Mizuoka, K., Matuhasi, T. and Fukuoka, Y. (1973). *In* "Immunopathology of the Skin: Labeled Antibody Studies," 1st ed. (Beutner, E. H., Chorzelski, T. P., Bean, S. F. and Jordon, R. E., eds.) Dowden, Hutchinson and Ross, Stroudsburg, Pennsylvania

McKinney, R. M., Spillane, J. and Pearce, G. W. (1964). *Anal Biochem* **9**, 474-76

Nisengard, R. J., Jablonska, S., Chorzelski, T. P., Blaszczyk, M., Jarrett, C. and Beutner, E. H. (1975). *Arch Derm* **111**, 1298-1300

Shu, S., Deng, J-S, Vetter, S. and Beutner, E. H. (1975). *Ann New York Acad Sci* **254**, 559 and 572

Shu, S., Nisengard, R. J., Hale, W. L. and Beutner, E. H. (1975). *J Lab Clin Med* **86**, 259-65

CHAPTER **II**

The State of the Art of Immunofluorescence Assays in Flow Cytometry

P. K. HORAN, Ph.D. and K. A. MUIRHEAD, Ph.D.

Table of Contents

1. Introduction

The application of flow cytometry to clinical immunology is a rapidly evolving topic for research. With this new technique, quantitative single particle analysis of fluorescence intensity and light-scatter intensity is possible at rates in excess of 50,000 particles or cells per minute. Some of the clinical applications include both humoral and cell-mediated immune assays. This article will describe the basic technology to familiarize the reader with the instrumentation (Horan and Wheeless, 1977; Herzenberg and Sweet, 1976). After the concepts of this instrumentation are covered, current and future applications of cell sorting to clinical immunology will be outlined.

The reader might ask, "What value is there in flow cytometry?" Current applications of fluorescence measurements in pathology appear to be finding their place without such sophisticated instrumentation. It should be noted that procedures utilizing sophisticated technology are not designed to replace current fluorescence procedures, but rather to augment them.

Flow cytometry has a number of attributes which make it very attractive. These include: 1) The method is capable of quantitatively measuring the fluorescence intensity from a single cell or particle; 2) Its sensitivity allows detection of as few as 3,000 fluorescein molecules per cell or particle; 3) Cells which possess the desired fluorescence intensity or light-scatter intensity can be recovered for further analysis; 4) Two-color fluorescence and light-scatter measurements can be made simultaneously on cells at rates up to 50,000 cells per minute; and 5) This methodology allows for both viable and sterile sorting.

To make fluorescence measurements on individual cells or particles, the suspension to be examined is introduced into the flow chamber of the flow cytometer (Figure 1) through a fine (capillary) sample tube. The particle-containing sample stream emitted from the flow chamber is surrounded by a

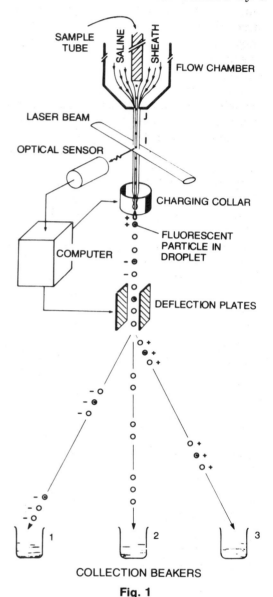

Fig. 1

SCHEMATIC DIAGRAM OF A FLOW CYTOMETER AND SORTER

Cells enter flow chamber through hypodermic needle and are centered by sheath saline in the sample stream. The exiting stream carries fluorescent particles from flow chamber through argon-ion laser beam. Two-color fluorescence emission and low angle light-scatter (1° - 20°) are recorded for each cell. Uniform droplets containing particles of interest can be charged electrostatically and sorted from the main stream.

laminar sheath of saline solution, resulting in a concentrically layered fluid stream which jets like water from a faucet from the flow chamber into the atmosphere. Particles are hydrodynamically confined to the center of the jet stream and are lined up like beads on a string.

After leaving the flow chamber, each particle in the stream passes through an argon-ion laser beam where simultaneous measurements of intensity of emitted fluorescent light and particle "size" (low angle light-scatter) can be made at rates of 50,000 to 100,000 cells or particles per minute. If it is determined that the particle at the laser beam-sample intersection is of interest, a time delay is initiated until the desired particle is at the droplet break-off point in the fluid jet.

At that point the sample stream is broken into small uniform droplets of saline, with a cell enclosed in every 30th droplet. As the droplets pass through the charging collar, the droplet containing the cell of interest and several on either side of it can be given either a positive or negative charge. The droplets continue to fall, passing through a pair of charged deflection plates which cause negatively charged drops (and particles of interest in them) to be deflected to the left into Beaker 1, and positively charged drops (containing other particles of interest) to be deflected to the right into Beaker 3. Uncharged droplets fall into Beaker 2. This important sorting feature permits the recovery of specific subpopulations from a complex mixture.

2. Cell-Mediated Immunity

A. T-Cell and B-Cell Analysis

The detection of T-cells and B-cells by flow cytometry can be accomplished using either fluorescence or light-scatter (Scher et al, 1976; Epstein et al, 1974; Goldberg et al, 1976). When using fluorescent techniques, specific antisera

for T- and B-cells must be obtained. It is possible to stain B- or T-cells separately using a fluorescein-conjugated antiserum and detect the positively fluorescent cells using a green sensitive photomultiplier tube. To permit simultaneous characterization of T-cells and B-cells, different fluorochromes must be conjugated to the anti-T and anti-B immunoglobulins. Fluorescein and rhodamine can be used for this purpose, although considerable optical and electronic signal processing is required for good results, since the excitation and emission spectra of these two fluorochromes are not especially well matched (Loken et al, 1977).

It is also possible to detect E-rosettes and/or EAC-rosettes on the basis of combined light-scatter and fluorescence measurements. If a population of rosettes and non-rosettes is stained with acridine orange, the lymphocytes take up stain and fluoresce, but neither human nor sheep erythrocytes fluoresce. It is then possible to require that only cells which fluoresce (or rosettes containing fluorescent cells) be further analyzed for light-scatter intensity.

The light-scatter range for non-rosetted lymphocytes can be established by measuring the light-scatter intensities of fluorescent cells in a population containing no rosettes. Rosetted lymphocytes will give rise to higher light-scatter intensities, being detected by the instrument simply as larger particles than non-rosettes. When the light-scatter profile of a population containing both rosettes and non-rosettes is compared with the profile obtained from non-rosettes, any increase in the high intensity light-scatter is therefore a direct measure of the rosette-forming cells within the population.

Thus, the detection of B- and T-cells can be achieved using flow cytometry. It is anticipated that in the future, with the development of more compatible fluorochromes than rhodamine and fluorescein, it will be possible to easily detect both B-cells and T-cells simultaneously using fluorochrome-conjugated anti-B and T-cell sera. This simultaneous detection of populations is extremely important when enumerating the null cell population.

B. Detection of Antigen Binding Cells

One of the newer areas in immunology is the study of functional ability of immune competent cells. While a few of these assays have begun to appear in the battery of immune testing, it is not yet understood how they can best be used. It appears that one of the more important functions of immune competent cells is the ability to recognize and bind to antigen. As we all know, recognition of antigen is the first step leading to the production of antibody and/or, possibly, cell-mediated killing. Thus, the ability to recognize a foreign antigen is an important component of immune competency.

Flow cytometry provides the ability to identify and quantitate not only the number of cells which recognize a particular antigen, but also the amount of antigen bound per cell (Julius and Herzenberg, 1974; Julius *et al*, 1972). The methodology used to achieve this goal involves fluoresceination of the antigen in question. After purification of a specific subset of immune competent cells (e.g. lymphocytes), the cells are exposed to the fluorescein conjugated antigen. The antigen binds to those cells that recognize it. The cells are then passed through a flow cytometer for an analysis of fluorescence intensity. Those cells which recognize and bind antigen are identifiable on the basis of their increased fluorescence intensity.

While this form of analysis is currently being utilized in research studies, it has not yet found its way into the battery of tests for clinical immunology. However, we must point out that this kind of assay provides an additional feature. Because

flow cytometers are capable of sorting cells, it would also be possible to sort the antigen binding cells into sterile beakers for further functional analysis.

Let us ask, for example, if it is possible for a given patient not only to bind antigen to immunocompetent cells, but also to produce antibody against a particular soluble protein antigen. After exposing the cells (lymphocytes) to fluorescein conjugated antigen, the cells which bind antigen would be sorted into beakers for further functional analysis. These cells could then be placed into Michelle-Dutton type cultures, and the ability to produce antibody against the specific antigen could be assessed.

C. Subpopulation Identification

One of the more interesting recent developments in flow cytometry is the ability to identify cells containing specific antigen markers on their surfaces. These analyses have been hampered by the fact that, typically, the antisera used are from rabbit or goat. These sera contain antibodies against a number of antigens on the cell surface. Hence, they are not monoclonal in the true sense of the word.

However, with the advent of xenogeneic myeloma-hybrid antibodies (Köhler and Milstein, 1975), it is now possible to make antibodies which are directed against a single protein entity on the surface of the cell. With this very powerful technique, it becomes possible to subclassify cells based purely on the antigen makeup on the surface of the cells. This kind of subclassification may become extremely useful in the identification and characterization of leukemia in humans. A number of workers are developing monospecific antisera which may help further classify the null cell population found in human leukemias (Greaves and Jannossy, 1975).

Similarly, it is also possible to use flow cytometry to identify specific subsets of cells which contain various receptor sites. Some of these receptor sites include Fc receptor, complement receptors, and red cell receptors. Using fluorescently tagged protein, such as fluorescein conjugated Fc, it now becomes possible to quantitatively and objectively ascertain the number of cells within the lymphocyte pool containing specific receptors. This kind of identification is in its infancy; it will be a number of years before these tests find clinical applicability.

D. Phagocytosis

Another functional attribute of immune competent cells is that of phagocytizing foreign materials. This function may be of clinical importance in assessing the total immune competence of a patient. Current assays measure the ingestion of bacteria or polystyrene microspheres. The particles, which may or may not be coded with antigen, are mixed with the cells to be tested in vitro. After an appropriate incubation time, the cells are examined, using a microscope to ascertain the extent of the phagocytic activity. In general, these assays can only be carried out on a limited basis because by microscopic observation only 200 to 500 cells can be examined per specimen. With such a small number of cells being examined it is difficult to accurately assess the number of particles phagocytized.

Using flow cytometry it is possible to rapidly examine several hundred thousand cells resulting in increased statistical reliability. The light-scatter intensity is examined for each cell as it passes through the laser beam. If a cell has phagocytized foreign particles, the light-scatter intensity, and therefore the profile, will be changed. As the cell phagocytizes an increasing number of particles, there is a corresponding increase in the light-scatter intensity. Thus, by flow cytometry it is not only possible to enumerate the percentage of the population capable of phagocytizing

a specific particle, but it is also possible to evaluate the extent of that phagocytosis (Leary).

E. Blastogenic Response

Another type of functional assay currently in use is the transformation assay. In this assay, purified immune competent cells are exposed to various mitogens. The mitogen treated cells and untreated control cells are incubated with tritiated thymidine. If the mitogen causes the immune competent cells to synthesize DNA, the tritiated thymidine is incorporated. Thus, the end point of the assay is the measuring of the increase in radioactivity per cell resulting from the exposure to a specific mitogen.

One of the major difficulties with this assay involves the fact that unstimulated control cultures may have a high-level background incorporation. Recent evidence suggests that this high background level incorporation may be due to recent infection giving rise to extensive repair synthesis. This will result in H^3-Thymidine incorporation even in the absence of de novo DNA synthesis. Thus, the ratio of counts incorporated by stimulated and unstimulated cells will be artificially low.

Using flow cytometry, a number of assays have been developed to assess the extent of the blastogenic response (Braunstein et al, 1976; Cram et al, 1976). Some of these assays use measurements of DNA content within cells. Other assays use the stain acridine orange to differentiate blast cells from normal untransformed cells. These assays do not suffer from the limitation that repair synthesis causes a change in control values because the amount of DNA per cell is not changed by repair synthesis.

3. Humoral Immunity

A. Determination of Specific Antibody Levels in Serum

Protein determinations of various immunoglobulins in serum have become a rather routine part of clinical immunology laboratories. While this is important, it is of equal importance to understand the specific antibody levels in serum. Several of the methods already in use depend upon a two-step process that involves not only antigen-antibody recognition, but also some secondary process such as agglutination, flocculation, etc.

Using a two-parameter cell sorter (Coulter Electronics, Hialeah, Florida), we have developed a new method for the detection of serum antibodies directed towards specific antigens which depends only on antigen-antibody rec-

ognition (Horan *et al*, 1979). This method is illustrated in Figure 2. Purified antigens are placed on polystyrene microspheres; in the example demonstrated, IgG_1 was adsorbed to 5μ spheres, IgG_2 was adsorbed to 11μ spheres, and IgG_3 adsorbed to 14μ spheres. After the primary antigen is adsorbed to the microspheres, they are then exposed to BSA. This results in reduced non-specific interactions between adsorbed IgG molecules and serum antibodies.

An aliquot containing all three sizes of IgG microspheres is then incubated with the patient's serum. If the patient has, for example, IgM antibodies which bind

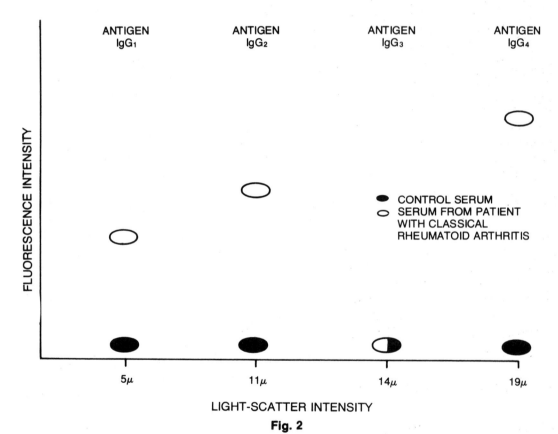

Fig. 2

IDEALIZED SIMULTANEOUS DETECTION OF IgM anti-IgG₁, IgG₂, IgG₃, AND IgG₄

IgG₁ would be adsorbed to 5µ polystyrene spheres, IgG₂ would be adsorbed to 11µ spheres, IgG₃ would be adsorbed to 14µ spheres, and IgG₄ would be adsorbed to 19µ spheres. Equal numbers of each size microsphere would be placed in patient's serum, washed and then reacted with fluorescein conjugated species anti-IgM. Using a flow cytometer, size (and therefore the adsorbed antigen) could be identified by light-scatter intensity. The corresponding fluorescence intensity (and therefore rheumatoid factor binding) could be measured using the photomultiplier tube.

to the IgG, the IgM will remain bound to the 5μ microspheres after they are washed free of patient serum. To detect the presence of the rheumatoid factor (IgM anti-IgG), fluorescein conjugated goat anti-μ is added. After washing away the unbound fluorescein conjugate, the microspheres are either fluorescent or non-fluorescent, depending upon whether IgM binds to the antigen initially placed on the microsphere.

To determine the fluorescence intensity, the microspheres are then passed through a two-parameter cell sorter. The cell sorter can identify the size of the particle on the basis of light-scatter intensity. Knowing the size of the particle, the investigator can identify the antigen bound to the microsphere. The light-scatter and fluorescence intensity of each microsphere are simultaneously recorded by the instrument. As seen in Figure 2, this kind of analysis results in a fingerprint profile, and when the results are compared to a normal control serum, the amount and type of autoimmune dysfunction can be identified.

Using this kind of methodology, we have shown that patients with rheumatoid arthritis who are seropositive have an IgM molecule or rheumatoid factor molecule which has a preference for binding to IgG_4. In order of intensity, the next highest level of binding is to IgG_2, then IgG_1, and last and lowest intensity is the IgM anti-IgG_3. We must point out that the IgM anti-IgG_3 level is the same as control serum.

B. Evaluation of Fluorescent Antibodies

The use of flow cytometry for the evaluation of fluorescently tagged antibodies is a major step in objectivity. The flow cytometer is exceedingly sensitive and can measure fluorescence intensities which are not visible in the microscope. Furthermore, flow cytometer measurements are not characterized by the same kind of subjectivity as measurements made with the human eye. While flow cytometry has its limitations, it is important to note that this method of valuation of fluorescent antibodies is a more objective method than others.

In a recent paper (Cram and Forslund, 1974), a simple method is outlined for the characterization of fluorescent antibodies. With this methodology, cells or microspheres containing the antigen to be evaluated are exposed to the fluorescein conjugated antibody in varying dilutions. The fluorescence intensity is then measured using the flow cytometer. By plotting the relative brightness or fluorescence intensity as a function of conjugate concentration and subtracting out the non-specific background fluorescence, an investigator can determine the concentration of maximum specificity.

4. Detection of Fetal Cells in Maternal Circulation

A. Fetal Erythrocytes

Clearly one of the major immunological problems confronting the clinician today involves the sensitization of an Rh negative mother by Rh positive fetal cells. This sensitization generally results in increased difficulty with subsequent pregnancies. To prevent this kind of complication, mothers with Rh incompatibility are very often injected with RhoGAM, but this type of injection may be needless for many mothers. Not only is it expensive, but in fact, the mother is being injected with a foreign protein. It would, therefore, be beneficial if the extent of the bleed of Rh positive cells into the maternal circulation could be characterized. If the level of Rh positive cells in the Rh negative mother is known, it may be possible to define a minimum threshold above which mothers should be injected with RhoGAM and below which mothers do not need to be injected with this foreign protein.

To achieve this goal, researchers are currently using fluorescein conjugated anti-D in an attempt to identify fetal cells in maternal circulation. If this procedure makes possible the identification of mothers at risk and differentiates these from others with low risk, it is very possible that this test will be implemented in the near future as a routine diagnostic test in clinical immunology. Currently, researchers at the University of Rochester (Doherty and Horan, 1978) are investigating this possibility using a TPS-1 cell sorter (Coulter Electronics, Hialeah, Florida).

B. Fetal Leukocytes

Another area of considerable interest is the identification and collection of fetal white cells from the maternal circulation. While it is true that amniocentesis does not pose a significant risk to the mother, it is also true that the cells obtained by amniocentesis are of poor culture quality. Many of these cells are exfoliated squamous cells and dead or dying lymphocytes.

If flow cytometry could achieve the recovery and identification of fetal lymphocytes in the maternal circulation, it would then be possible to culture these cells for karyotyping. Fetal cells sorted from the maternal circulation could be exposed to mitogen and colchicine and after the appropriate time the mitoses prepared for genetic analysis. This research is currently going on in the United States and England, and the results of those efforts are soon to be published (Herzenberg *et al*, 1979).

5. Summary

The application of flow cytometry to clinical immunology is an area of expanding interest. Because of the method's extreme sensitivity it is of paramount importance that the reagents used in any flow cytometric assay be fully characterized. Ideally only $F(ab')_2$ antibodies having monoclonal specificities should be used. Use of antisera produced in animals should be considered suboptimal, as cross-reacting or sub-major species not detectable by other methods may give rise to unacceptable background levels using flow cytometry. With the availability of new methods for producing monoclonal antibodies, the ideal of monoclonal specificity is much more attainable.

A major concern with regard to regulation of flow cytometric assays is that they should not be constrained to initiate current methods. Cells classified into discrete states using microscopic morphometric analysis may not yield exactly the same classifications when analyzed by flow cytometry. Increased sensitivity, quantifiability, and statistical accuracy possible using flow cytometry mean that this method may yield different information from currently available assays, and therein lies its great potential. Flow cytometry can be expected to yield information capable of augmenting current methods, but requiring it to replace them by yielding identical information will simply hamper its development.

6. References

Braunstein, J. D., Good, R. A., Hansen, J. A., Sharpless, T. K. and Melamed, M. R. (1976). *J Histochem Cytochem* **24**, 378

Cram, L. S. and Forslund, J. C. (1974). *Immunochem* **11**, 667

Cram, L. S., Gomez, E. R., Thoen, C. O., Forslund, J. C. and Jett, J. H. (1976). *J Histochem Cytochem* **24**, 383

Doherty, R. A. and Horan, P. K. (1978). *Am J Dis Child* **132**, 556

Epstein, L. B., Kreth, H. W. and Herzenberg, L. A. (1974). *Cell Immunol* **12**, 407-21

Goldberg, N. H., Kenady, D. E., Super, B. S. and Chretien, P. B. (1976). *J Immunol Meth* **12**, 9-17

Greaves, M. F. and Jannossy, G. (1976). *In* "In Vitro Methods in Cell-Mediated and

Tumor Immunity" (Bloom, B. R. and David, J. R., eds.) p. 89, Academic Press, New York

Herzenberg, L. A., Bianchi, D. W., Schröder, J., Conn, H. M. and Iveson, G. M. (1979). *Proc Nat Acad Sci* **76**, 1453-55

Herzenberg, L. A. and Sweet, R. G. (1976). *Sci Am* **234**, 108

Horan, P. K., Schenk, E. A., Abraham, G. and Kloszewski, E. (1979). *In* "Immunoassays in the Clinical Laboratory" (Nakamura, R. M., Dito, W. R. and Tucker, E. S., eds.) Alan Liss, Inc., New York

Horan, P. K. and Wheeless, L. L. (1977). *Science* **198**, 149

Julius, M. and Herzenberg, L. A. (1974). *J Exp Med* **140**, 904

Julius, M. H., Masuda, T. and Herzenberg, L. A. (1972). *Proc Nat Acad Sci* **69**, 1934

Köhler, G. and Milstein, C. (1975). *Nature* **256**, 495

Leary, J. F. Personal communication

Loken, M. R., Parks, D. R. and Herzenberg, L. A. (1977). *J Histochem Cytochem* **25**, 899

Scher, I., Sharrow, S. O., Wistar, R., Asofsky, R. and Paul, W. E. (1976). *J Exp Med* **144**, 494-506

CHAPTER III

Future Trends and Applications of Immunofluorescent Techniques

R. M. NAKAMURA, M.D.

Table of Contents

1. Introduction

Most fluorophores or fluorescent compounds are organic compounds with a ring structure. When the compound absorbs light, there is an excitation of electrons which oscillate in resonance. With the absorption of light of shorter wavelength, the energy can be emitted in the form of light of longer wavelength with a short time lapse between absorption and emission of light. The approximate time interval between absorption of energy and emission of fluorescence is less than 10^{-9} seconds.

The sensitivity of fluorimetric methods can now be refined to detect substances at concentrations of 10^{-15} M. Advances have been made possible by recent improvements in instrumentation and the employment of unique substrate reactants with different immunochemical and enzymatic reactions.

This discussion will be limited to fluid phase methods and will not include methods involving measurement of immunochemical reactions on cells or large particles.

2. Increase or Decrease of Hapten Fluorescence by Antibody

In the fluorescence quenching method, the binding of a chromophoric hapten by antibody causes a marked decrease of antibody tryptophane fluorescence (Parker, 1973). Smith (1977) has described an enhancement fluoroimmunoassay of thyroxine. A fluorescent derivative of thyroxine (T_4), whose fluorescence was enhanced when bound to anti-T_4 serum, was used in the assay method. The assay involves a short incubation step following the mixing of the sample, labeled T_4, and specific antiserum with subsequent measurement of the fluorescence enhancement (Figure 1). An Aminco-Bowman SPF fluorimeter was used to measure the degree of fluorescence.

Fluorescein-T_4 conjugate is not an efficient fluorophore since there is intramolecular quenching of the fluorescein fluorophore by the iodine atoms of the iodothyronine portion of the T_4

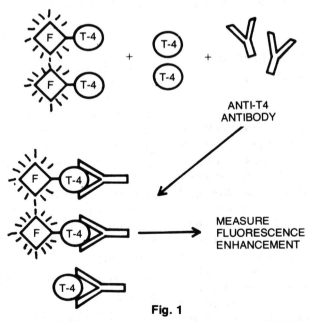

ANTI-T4
ANTIBODY

MEASURE
FLUORESCENCE
ENHANCEMENT

Fig. 1

ENHANCEMENT FLUOROIMMUNOASSAY OF THYROXINE

With permission—Nakamura, R.M. (1977)

molecule. Such iodine-containing molecules are efficient quenchers of fluorescence. However, when specific antibody binds to T₄, there is enhancement of fluorescence to a maximum of 3.9-fold. This enhancement is best explained in terms of inhibition of quenching when the iodothyronine moiety becomes interlocked into the combining site of the specific anti-T₄ antibody. This assay can be performed with a conventional fluorimeter.

One of the disadvantages of using conventional fluorimetric instrumentation is the variability of levels of intrinsic serum fluorescence in the patient samples. The assay procedure requires either a reliable technique to remove background interference of the intrinsic serum fluorescence or special instrumentation to increase the sensitivity and specificity of the assay. With use of a conventional fluorimeter, the technique as published is less sensitive than standard radioimmunoassay methods for T₄; however, removal of the variable background serum sample fluorescence would allow sufficient sensitivity to measure total T₄ levels in clinical patients.

3. Polarization of Antigen or Hapten Fluorescence by Antibody

Light can be resolved with a polarizing lens or prism into rays with their electrical vectors in a single plane. Fluorescent solutions which are excited with vertically polarized or natural light emit partially polarized fluorescence as viewed at right angles to the incident beam. Polarization of fluorescence is due to the fixed relationship between molecular orientation and the absorption and emission of fluorescence. Specific regions of the fluorescent molecule are concerned with absorption and emission, and are termed absorption and emission oscillators. They become oscillating electrical dipoles during activation of fluorescence (Parker, 1973).

This method is useful for the measurement of small fluorescent haptens and for fluorescent protein antigens combined with antibody. Most of the published fluorescence polarization methods involve labeled antigen (Dandliker and de Saussure, 1970; Dandliker et al, 1973; Dandliker et al, 1978). The sensitivity of the method is dependent upon the binding affinity of the antibody; concentrations can be assayed at one nanogram per ml or less of human chorionic gonadotrophin (Dandliker et al, 1973).

Fluorescent polarization methods are of limited use in the clinical laboratory since no change in polarization has been observed in studies with fluorescent labeled antibody or antibody fragments (Dandliker and de Saussure, 1970; Dandliker et al, 1973).

4. Heterogeneous Immunoassays with Fluorescent Labeled Antibody

There are basically two types of assays (Aalberse, 1973; Burgett et al, 1977a; Burgett et al, 1977b; Blanchard and Gardner, 1978); most which are commercially available utilize a solid phase antigen or antibody system. An assay can be developed either as a competitive or non-competitive type. The method selected is often dependent on the degree of sensitivity and specificity desired. Current assays use a conventional fluorimeter and the sensitivity of the method is often limited to about 10^{-8} to 10^{-9} molar concentrations of the antigen assayed.

A. Heterogeneous Solid Phase Antigen Assay

A solid phase antigen competes with free antigen and labeled antibody. After equilibrium has been reached, the fluorescent labeled antibody attached to the solid phase is measured. This procedure requires a washing step to separate bound and unbound labeled antibody.

B. Heterogeneous Solid Phase Antibody Assay

In this procedure, unlabeled antibody to the antigen is adsorbed or covalently linked to a solid phase. The antigen and labeled specific antibody may be added sequentially or simultaneously, as competitive inhibition technique. The latter competitive inhibition type of assay is termed non-homogeneous solid phase antibody-inhibition fluorescent immunoassay. Many of the serum proteins have been measured by these solid phase antibody methods.

Commercially available kits for assay of certain serum proteins, such as IgG, IgM, IgA, C3, and C4, are available from International Diagnostic Technology, Inc., Santa Clara, California, and Bio-Rad Laboratories, Richmond, California. In the assays for C3 and C4, sensitivity is in the range of 125 nanograms/ml for C3, and 150 nanograms/ml for C4 (Burgett *et al*, 1977a; 1977b). The commercially available immunofluorescent procedures for IgG and IgM quantitation have been compared with the radial immunodiffusion values. There was good agreement of the immunofluorescent quantitative values for IgG and IgA concentrations; however, the IgM values obtained by immunofluorescent assays were significantly lower than the radial immunodiffusion values (Blanchard and Gardner, 1978).

5. Fluorescence Immunoassay by Internal Reflection Spectroscopy

A new immunoassay technique (Kronick and Little, 1975) has been described which uses the total internal reflection of light to excite the fluorescence of fluorescein labeled antibody which is bound to a hapten-protein conjugate adsorbed on a quartz plate in the antibody solution. The presence of any free hapten in solution reduces the amount of labeled antibody bound to the surface of the quartz plate. The fluorescence of the surface of the quartz plate is measured by a special technique in which only the fluorescent molecules at the *surface* of the quartz plate are measured, and the labeled antibody in the free solution is not activated. The excitation beam is reflected at a *special angle* so that only the solid phase is activated, thus *eliminating the separation step of bound and unbound labeled antibody.*

Kronick and Little (1975) have successfully measured morphine at a concentration of 2×10^{-7} M by this method, which is simple and rapid, exhibiting a high degree of intrinsic sensitivity and specificity. Antigen or hapten-protein conjugate is bound onto the quartz surface in contact with the solution under test (Figure 2). Blue light from a helium-cadmium laser strikes the quartz-water interface at an angle of θ greater than the critical angle so it undergoes total internal reflection. Thus, the blue light penetrates only minimally into the solution for a depth of only a few angstroms. The fluorescein conjugated antibody which binds to the antigen on the surface of the quartz plate is excited by the evanescent wave of the excitation laser light and fluoresces, while the conjugated antibody in the solution beyond the evanescent wave region of the excitation light is not excited and, consequently, does not fluoresce. The instrument has a photomultiplier tube enabling a view of the fluorescence on the quartz surface. The filter between the photomultiplier and the quartz surface allows only the green fluorescent light to reach the photomultiplier tube.

In the test method with antigen coated

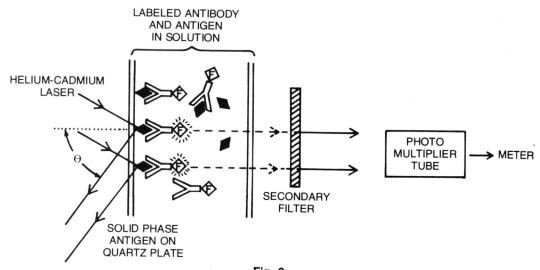

Fig. 2

SOLID PHASE ANTIGEN FLUORESCENCE IMMUNOASSAY
BY INTERNAL REFLECTION SPECTROSCOPY

With permission—Nakamura, R.M. (1977)

quartz, there are initially no specific conjugated antibodies on the plate, and as the reaction proceeds to equilibrium, fluorescent antibodies will bind to the quartz surface. The concentration of fluorescent antibody on the quartz surface will decrease in proportion to the concentration of hapten antigen in the competing unknown sample. The sensitivity of this method can be enhanced by using solid phase unlabeled specific antibody with a sandwich technique involving fluorescent labeled specific antibody. The technique can be used to assay for *multiple constituents* in the *same sample* by placement of different antigens or antibodies on specific spots of the quartz plate. The solution would also contain multiple types of conjugated specific antibodies to the various constituents assayed. The same fluorescein label may be conjugated to the various different specific antibodies. However, the system would require the scanning and quantitation of the fluorescent emission of the multiple spots on the quartz plate (Kronick and Little, 1976).

This system has certain disadvantages, notably, those of background non-specific fluorescence and scatter of light. However, the sensitivity of the method can be enhanced more than 10^{-6} times by using the modified cross correlation phase fluorescence instrument described below. Use of this instrument would increase the sensitivity of fluorescence measurements to concentrations of less than 10^{-12} molar concentrations with a range of sensitivity equal to, or greater than, most sensitive radioimmunoassay procedures.

6. Homogeneous Fluorescent Excitation Transfer Immunoassay

This is a general immunochemical method for assay of haptens and proteins (Ullman *et al*, 1976). The assay has been devised and applied to analysis of morphine, a morphine-albumin conjugate, and human IgG immunoglobulin.

The fluorescence excitation transfer method employs two labels. Fluorescein is used as a donor fluorescer and the rhodamine label is used as the acceptor or quencher. Fluorescein isothiocyanate has a maximum emission of 525nm and tetramethyl or tetraethyl rhodamine has a strong absorption peak at 525nm. Therefore, when FITC labeled antigen and rhodamine labeled antibody bind, there is a *quenching* of FITC fluorescence when the two labels are within a distance of 50 to 100 angstroms.

Two variants of the method were studied (Figure 3). In the first, the antigen (Ag) was labeled with fluorescein (F) and the antibody (Ab) was labeled with rhodamine (R). This method may be referred to as the direct antigen labeling method. When using fluorescein and rhodamine as the fluorescer and quencher, the average distance between them must be sufficient to permit dipole-dipole coupled excitation energy

1.) $Ag + (F - Ag) \cdot (R - Ab) \leftrightarrows Ag \cdot R - Ab + \substack{F \\ - Ab}$

2.) $Ag + F \cdot Ab + R - Ab \leftrightarrows (R - Ab)_n - Ag(F - Ab)_m$ MULTIVALENT

Fig. 3

FLUORESCENT EXCITATION TRANSFER IMMUNOASSAY

transfer within the antigen-antibody complex. In the assay procedure for quantitation of antigen in unknown samples, the unlabeled antigen would compete for the rhodamine labeled antibody and reduce available binding sites with reduction in the amount of quenching.

The second method (Figure 3) is similar to the first except that the antigen is labeled *indirectly* by employing a fluorescein labeled antibody. This method is useful for assay of antigen with multivalent antigenic determinants. Separate portions of specific antibody are labeled with fluorescein and rhodamine, respectively. The admixture of differently labeled fluorescein tagged antibody and rhodamine labeled antibody would reduce the intensity of the fluorescer by adjusting the ratio and amount of donor and acceptor so they react in close proximity to permit energy transfer. A definite disadvantage of the indirect labeling method is that immunochemically purified antibodies are required so as to avoid excessive fluorescence background due to non-specific fluorescer labeled proteins. These assays have a potential sensitivity in the 100 picomole range. The advantages over heterogeneous assays include speed, avoidance of the separation step, and stability of the reagents.

7. Direct Antigen Labeling Fluorescent Excitation Transfer Immunoassay

This technique was studied in the assay of morphine (Figure 4). Addition of increasing amounts of rhodamine labeled anti-morphine to a fixed concentration of morphine-fluorescein will pro-

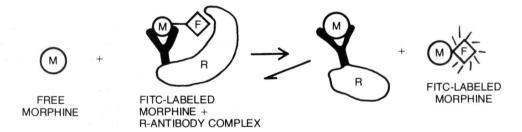

FREE MORPHINE + FITC-LABELED MORPHINE + R-ANTIBODY COMPLEX → + FITC-LABELED MORPHINE

Fig. 4

HOMOGENEOUS FLUORESCENT EXCITATION TRANSFER IMMUNOASSAY FOR MORPHINE

With permission—Nakamura, R.M. (1977)

duce decreases in fluorescence intensity which will approach a minimum value with excess antibody. A maximum quenching of 72% was observed with an excess of specific antibody labeled with 15 molecules of rhodamine.

In the studies by Ullman *et al* (1976), the fluorescence measurements were made with a Perkin-Elmer MPF-2A spectrofluorometer equipped with Baird-Atomic B-4 and B-5 fluorescein filters. The excitation light was at 470nm and the emission maximum was found near 520nm. The direct antigen labeling method has been applied to assays for human IgG, using fluorescein labeled IgG and rabbit anti-human IgG labeled with rhodamine.

8. Indirect Antigen Labeling Fluorescent Excitation Transfer Immunoassay

This assay method is useful for antigens with multiple determinants and requires an immunochemically purified preparation of fluorescein labeled antibody. The assay has been applied to a hapten, such as morphine, by employing morphine-albumin conjugates (albumin-M_{30}) which have 30 molecules of morphine bound to one molecule of albumin. The assay was sensitive for albumin-M_{30} and codeine to a level of one nanomole.

Similarly, an indirect assay was developed for human IgG. Ullman *et al*

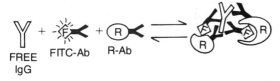

Fig. 5

HOMOGENEOUS FLUORESCENT EXCITATION TRANSFER IMMUNOASSAY FOR IgG WITH PAIRED LABEL ANTIBODY TO IgG

With permission—Nakamura, R.M. (1977)

(1976) labeled separate portions of immunochemically purified antibodies to human IgG with fluorescein and rhodamine, respectively (Figure 5). The sensitivity of the assay for human IgG was below 100 picomoles.

9. Antigen Labeled Fluorescence Protection Assay

In this assay, the protein antigen is labeled with fluorescein and then reacted with specific antibody to the antigen (Ullman, 1978a). The antigen-specific antibody will sterically inhibit the reaction of the antibody specific for fluorescein which, in turn, will quench the fluorescence of fluorescein when it binds to the fluorophore. The specific anti-fluorescein may be coupled to dextran or complexed with antibodies to the anti-fluorescein to increase the size and decrease the ability to interact with the fluorescein coupled to the surface of the antigen within a small space. The procedure may be used to assay for antibody to the antigen or the antigen concentration in a homogeneous system.

Ullman (1978a; 1978b) used the technique for assay of serum T-4 levels, and also as a test for anti-cardiolipin antibody similar to a serologic screening test for syphilis. Liposomes with the cardiolipin antigen are labeled with fluorescein. When the fluorescein-labeled antigen is first reacted with anti-cardiolipin antigen, the antibody-labeled antigen complex in turn will inhibit, by steric hindrance, the reaction of the fluorescein-labeled antigen with anti-fluorescein antibody. The cardiolipin antigen concentration measured is directly related to the degree of fluorescence observed in the reaction.

The assay for T-4 involves fluorescein-labeled T-4 complexed with low affinity anti-fluorescein antibody which decreases the fluorescence of fluorescein. When anti-T-4 is added, the anti-

T-4 reacts with the fluorescein-labeled T-4 and pulls it away from the specific anti-fluorescein antibody, resulting in an increase in fluorescence.

In the assay of serum samples with high concentrations of T-4, the anti-T-4 will react with the T-4, and the fluorescence will be decreased since anti-fluorescein will remain complexed to the labeled T-4. The assay shows very little interference with background serum proteins. It is feasible to measure T-4 levels in clinical samples in a sensitive and reproducible fashion.

10. Homogeneous Reactant-Labeled Fluorescent Immunoassay

This assay has been adapted to measure gentamicin levels (Burd *et al*, 1977). In the gentamicin assay, gentamicin is coupled to B-galactosyl umbelliferone to form a non-fluorescent substrate. The free B-galactosyl umbelliferone-gentamicin conjugate will react with the enzyme B-galactosidase to form a fluores-

cent product. However, when the B-galactosyl umbelliferone-gentamicin is combined with specific antibody, the linking of specific antibody by steric hindrance will not allow cleavage of the conjugate-antibody complex by B-galactosidase (Figure 6).

The procedure does not require a separation step and is a sensitive homogeneous assay. The rate of production of fluorescence was proportional to the gentamicin concentration, and the fluorescent assay yielded values which were comparable to those of a radioimmunoassay for gentamicin in clinical serum samples. The fluorescent assay requires $1\mu l$ of serum and can easily detect levels of gentamicin of less than $1\mu g/ml$. The procedure was completed in two to three minutes, and the fluorescence rate reaction was measured with an Aminco-Bowman spectrophotofluorometer equipped with temperature control for the sample compartment.

The principle of homogeneous reactant-labeled fluorescent immunoassay has been used to detect specific binding proteins (Burd *et al*, 1977). For example,

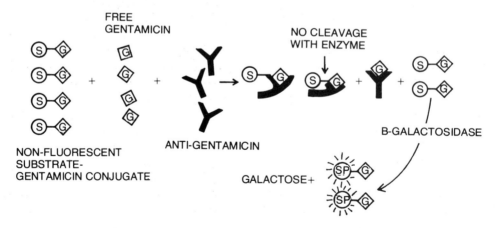

Fig. 6

HOMOGENEOUS REACTANT LABELED
FLUORESCENT IMMUNOASSAY
FOR GENTAMICIN

With permission—Nakamura, R.M. (1977)

biotin was coupled directly to umbelliferone through an ester bond. Hydrolysis of the non-fluorescent ester with an esterase, e.g. porcine esterase, yielded fluorescent products, and the reaction rate was related quantitatively to the conjugate concentration. When the conjugated ligand of biotin was bound to the specific protein binder avidin, they were not active as substrates. Thus, the technique can be used to assay for specific binding proteins as well as to measure levels of free ligand.

11. Modified Instrumentation for Increased Sensitivity of Fluorescent Measurements

There have been many innovative approaches to decreasing the background fluorescence and increasing the sensitivity of specific fluorescence measurements so that there is a marked increase in the specific signal-to-background ratio. Some of these methods are discussed below.

A. Pulse light source for quantitation of fluorescence

One can use a pulse excitation light source in the nanosecond range to activate the specific fluorescent compounds and reduce background. The specific emission light can be amplified and measured. Compounds which require a longer time interval of excitation would not be activated; such compounds may increase the background in conventional fluorimeters. A strobe light source at 3400°K activates the fluorescein labeled sample for less than 1/10,000 of a second, and the secondary fluorescent beam is passed through a filter to a photomultiplier system to quantitatively measure the total amount of light emitted at 525nm. Hans Nollar (1977) has shown evidence that the technique can be applied to detect hepatitis B antigen in serum samples with a sensitivity and specificity comparable to standard radioimmunoassay procedures.

The method uses segments of nylon mesh impregnated with patient serum samples fixed with acetone and water solution and then reacted with specific fluorescein isothiocyanate labeled anti-hepatitis B antibody. The nylon mesh segment is then washed with buffer solution, the specific fluorescent reactant on the nylon strip is eluted with an alkaline wash, and the fluorescence of the eluate is measured in the instrument with the pulse light source.

B. Cross correlation phase fluorimeter

The cross correlation phase fluorimeter can be used to directly determine fluorescence lifetimes of subnanoseconds (Little, 1978). The instrument employs complex electro-optical frequency measurements such that the half life of fluorescein isothiocyanate emission (about 10^{-9} seconds) can be measured. The cross correlation phase fluorimeter can be combined with internal reflectance spectroscopy (Kronick and Little, 1975) to increase the sensitivity and specificity of fluorescence measurements so that concentrations of substance of less than picomolar concentrations can be accurately measured. This instrument is capable of measuring a wide spectral range with an extremely high degree of sensitivity.

A laser beam is passed through a birefringent crystal under conditions producing a high frequency pulsating narrow band which is adjusted to obtain optimum phase lag of the fluorescence and excitation emissions.

The sensitivity of the instrument is increased if the photo current produced by the fluorescence is mixed with a voltage near, but not equal to, the modulating light frequency and the phase is measured in the amplified difference signal. An alternative technique is to transpose the original high frequency to a desired lower frequency and still main-

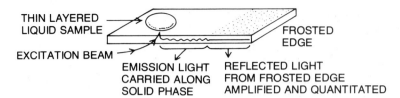

THIN LAYERED LIQUID SAMPLE

EXCITATION BEAM →

FROSTED EDGE

EMISSION LIGHT CARRIED ALONG SOLID PHASE

REFLECTED LIGHT FROM FROSTED EDGE AMPLIFIED AND QUANTITATED

Fig. 7

HOMOGENEOUS IMMUNOFLUORESCENT
ASSAY BY SOLID PHASE
REFLECTANCE

With permission—Nakamura, R.M. (1977)

tain a precise relationship in order to increase sensitivity of measurement.

W. A. Little (1978) has been developing a method combining solid phase reflectance with the cross correlation phase fluorimeter. In this method (Figure 7), antigen can be covalently linked to the surface of the glass slide; the specific fluorescent tagged antibody and antigen is in solution and reacted with an antigen linked spot on the glass slide. The slide is placed in an enclosed box and the excitation beam activates the fluorescent antibody conjugates on the surface of the glass slide. The emission of fluorescent light is carried along the solid phase of the glass slide, then reflected from the frosted edge, and amplified and quantitated with the specially-adapted instrument utilizing principles of cross correlation phase fluorimetry. The instrument is designed to measure the solid phase fluorescence and minimize the background interference of excitation in the free solution allowing for a homogeneous assay.

If one were to place many different antigen spots on the same slide and use a solution containing many different types of specific antibodies, by scanning the slide one would be able to quantitate and assay for multiple constituents in the same serum sample on the single slide.

12. Summary

Immunofluorescent assays are cur-

rently being developed which have great future promise and potential. The fluorescent assay can be developed to have equal or greater sensitivity than current sensitive radioimmunoassay procedures.

The advantages of immunofluorescent assays are:

a. Stability of reagents

b. High sensitivity and speed of measurement

c. Adaptability to automation

d. Homogeneous systems can be developed for complex protein antigens. (It is difficult to develop homogeneous assays for protein antigen by immunoenzyme methods.)

e. Immunofluorescent systems can be developed to rapidly quantitate multiple constituents in a single specimen sample.

On the other hand, the disadvantages of such procedures are:

a. Special expensive instrumentation is often required to reduce background interference.

b. Special immunochemically purified labeled antibody reagents must be prepared and standardized to obtain the desired sensitivity, specificity, and precision.

13. References

Aalberse, R. C. (1973). *Clin Chim Acta* **48**, 109

Blanchard, G. C. and Gardner, R. (1978). *Clin Chem* **24**, 808

Burd, J. F., Carrico, R. J., Fetter, M. C., Buckler, R. T., Johnson, R. D., Boguslaski, R. C. and Christner, J. E. (1977). *Anal Biochem* **77**, 56

Burd, J. F., Wong, R. C., Feeney, J. E.,

Carrico, R. J. and Boguslaski, R. C. (1977). *Clin Chem* **23**, 1402

Burgett, M. W., Fairfield, S. J. and Monthony, J. F. (1977a). *Clin Chim Acta* **78**, 277

Burgett, M. W., Fairfield, S. J. and Monthony, J. F. (1977b). *J Immunol Meth* **16**, 211

Dandliker, W. B., Dandliker, J., Levison, S. A., Kelly, R. J., Hicks, A. N. and White, J. U. (1978). *In* "Methods in Enzymology," Vol. 48 (Hirs, C. H. W. and Timasheff, S. N., eds.) Academic Press, New York

Dandliker, W. B., Kelly, R. J., Dandliker, J., Farquhar, J. and Levin, J. (1973). *Immunochem* **10**, 219

Dandliker, W. B. and de Saussure, V. A. (1970). *Immunochem* **7**, 799

Kronick, M. N. and Little, W. A. (1975). *J Immunol Meth* **8**, 235

Kronick, M. N. and Little, W. A. (1976). U.S. Patent #3,939,350

Little, W. A. (1978). Dept. of Physics, Stanford Univ., Palo Alto, CA

Nakamura, R. M. (1979). *In* "Immunoassays in the Clinical Laboratory" (Nakamura, R. M., Dito, W. R. and Tucker, E. S., eds.) Alan Liss, Inc., New York

Nollar, H. (1977). Personal communication

Parker, C. W. (1973). *In* "Handbook of Experimental Immunology," Vol. 1 (Weir, D. M., ed.) chap. 14, Blackwell Scientific, London

Smith, D. S. (1977). *FEBS Letter* **77**, 25

Spencer, R. D. and Weber, G. (1968). *Ann NY Acad Sci* **158**, 361

Ullman, E. F. (1978a). *Clin Chem* **24**, 973

Ullman, E. F. (1978b). Syva Corp., patent pending, personal communication

Ullman, E. F., Schwartzberg, M. and Rubenstein, K. D. (1976). *J Biol Chem* **251**, 4172

PART IV

DIAGNOSTIC IMMUNOLOGY

CHAPTER **I**

State of the Art of Procedures for Cellular Immunity

B. P. BARNA, Ph.D., S. D. DEODHAR, M.D., Ph.D.

Table of Contents

1. Introduction

Recognition of the complex cellular basis of the immune response from a historical standpoint has been an exciting and relatively recent occurrence. Analyses of cellular immunity and identification of cell populations have led to a better understanding of immune deficiency syndromes, autoimmune disease, transplantation, malignancy, infectious disease, certain hypersensitivity states, and problems of aging.

Cellular immunity techniques in vitro are loosely comprised of two general types of assays: those dealing with identification and quantitation of leukocytes and those assessing cellular function. Functional assays measure such lymphocyte responses as proliferation, secretion of lymphokines, and cytotoxicity. Monocyte function, such as phagocytosis or the response to chemotactic stimuli, may also be evaluated. At the present time, clinical use of these assays is limited by their requirement for somewhat delicate and time-consuming procedures and, consequently, their inability to provide immediate results.

With the exception of some types of immune deficiency, assays of cellular immune function are not diagnostic in nature. They are valuable primarily as indicators of total immunologic competence in response to changing clinical conditions. Measurements of cellular immunity may be helpful in judging the efficacy of immunosuppressive drugs in autoimmune disease or transplantation, or in evaluation of immunotherapy regimens in cancer or immune deficiency states.

All of the cellular immunology assays to be discussed here are performed in the Department of Immunopathology of the Cleveland Clinic Foundation, and the majority are offered as a routine clinical service. Some techniques, such as those dealing with macrophage function, are in the developmental stage.

2. Quality Control and Cellular Immunity Testing

The development of clinical methodology in cell-mediated immunity has been enhanced by the adoption of many aseptic culture techniques derived from virology and microbiology laboratories. In addition, innovative quality control procedures have been designed to ensure maintenance of optimum culture conditions and thus promotion of activity by responding immunologic cell populations.

One of the most important prerequisites for performance of cellular immunity assays is freshly-drawn viable leukocytes. Manipulation of lymphoid cells must be done gently, with minimum trauma, to retain surface or functional characteristics. Each laboratory reagent, including serum, medium, or mitogen, requires pretesting with viable cells before its use in clinical assays. Equipment, such as incubators and radioactivity counters, must be monitored daily, with major maintenance chores done professionally every six months. Techniques of cell preservation in liquid nitrogen storage are being tested with the hope that positive or negative quality control specimens can be stored and ready to thaw for testing at any time, thus obviating the necessity for fresh control blood samples.

Reference standard cell preparations are not available to the clinical cellular immunology laboratory and access to a reference "cell bank" would be highly desirable. Establishment of such a facility, however, would entail innumerable problems and would necessitate the development of reliable methods for preservation and transport of viable lymphocytes with stable defined functional properties and surface markers.

3. Identification of Lymphocyte Subpopulations

Quantitation of lymphocytes is accomplished by analysis of surface membrane markers on living cells and involves a series of lengthy and complex procedures. One of the most important uses of such procedures is in the diagnosis of lymphoproliferative disease where malignant cell type may influence selection of therapy. For example, more aggressive therapeutic regimens are prescribed for T-cell than for "null" cell acute leukemias (Whiteside and Rowlands, 1977).

T-cells are recognized by their capacity to form rosettes with neuraminidase-treated sheep red blood cells (E); the percentage of E-rosette-forming T-cells in our laboratory is normally in the range of 70% to 80%. The presence of surface immunoglobulin on B-cells is identified by immunofluorescent microscopy utilizing fluorescein-labeled antibody to human immunoglobulins. Normal range for immunoglobulin-bearing cells is 10% to 20%. Antibody and complement-coated sheep red blood cells are used to detect B-cell C3 receptors which are present on approximately 15% to 27% of normal lymphocytes. Use of a fluorescence activated cell sorter (FACS) for more objective and reliable identification of lymphocytes is in the developmental stage. Fluorescein-labeled C3 and antibody to human immunoglobulins are currently being tested for B-cell quantitation, and efforts are being made to develop T-cell antiserum.

Lymphocyte membrane receptors to specific viruses are also under investigation by means of a rosette assay in which lymphocytes are allowed to bind to measles-infected epithelial cells. This assay, which was developed by Levy et al (1976) at Duke University, has shown some promise in differentiating multiple sclerosis patients from those with other neurologic diseases. Lymphocytes from multiple sclerosis patients appear to possess large numbers of receptors for measles antigens, whereas lymphocytes

from normal or other patient groups do not. However, the clinical significance of this assay remains to be determined.

4. Proliferation Assays

Since the advent of the multiple automatic sample harvester (MASH), lymphocyte transformation testing has become a relatively simple microprocedure in which lymphocytes proliferate and incorporate radiolabeled thymidine in response to either mitogens or specific antigens. Incubation times for this assay range from four to six days, depending upon the reagent used. Mitogens commonly employed are phytohemagglutinin, concanavalin A, and pokeweed mitogen, which primarily stimulate T-cell subpopulations in a nonspecific fashion; B-cells also respond with T-cell help. As yet, we have not found a mitogen as specific for stimulation of human B-lymphocytes as lipopolysaccharide is for murine B-cells.

Depression of mitogen-induced lymphocyte proliferation has been noted in a number of clinical disorders, including lymphoproliferative and other malignant diseases, viral infections, sarcoidosis, and certain immune deficiency syndromes. In addition, steroids, cytotoxic drugs, or aspirin may have adverse effects upon cell reactivity.

Lymphocyte proliferation in vitro may occur in response to specific antigens to which the donor has been previously sensitized. Common recall antigens such as candida and PPD are used to test for the presence of immunologic memory. Lymphocyte transformation may also be applied in testing for hypersensitivity to metals, such as nickel or beryllium, or to various drugs, especially antibiotics. This assay has not been shown to have predictive value, however, and is therefore not suitable as a screening test. Detection of drug allergy by this test is also complicated by a high frequency of false negative results due to inherent technical difficulties.

5. Assays of Secretory Function

The most common assay for a lymphocyte secretory function is the migration inhibition test. In this assay, antigen stimulates secretion of a lymphokine which exerts an inhibitory effect on random leukocyte movement. We prefer the direct method in which mononuclear cells from peripheral blood are placed in capillary tubes and then exposed to specific antigens for 24 hours. The degree of migration from the capillary tubes is calculated after migration areas have been projected onto paper and the paper images have been weighed. Although secretion of migration inhibitory factor (MIF) in response to specific recall antigens may also be measured indirectly by using guinea pig peritoneal macrophages, performance of the direct test is more convenient for a clinical laboratory. The migration inhibition assay is technically difficult, however, and requires stringent pretesting of antigens at various doses to minimize the possibility of false positive results due to antigen toxicity. Extremely dilute concentrations of antigen may enhance migration and thus give rise to false negative results.

Investigation of suppressor factor secretion by T-cells is also underway in our department. Suppressor factors are recognized by their ability to cause reduction of pokeweed mitogen-induced immunoglobulin synthesis, and although such assays are presently on a research basis, they may show promise for clinical use.

6. Cytotoxicity Assays

Interpretation of studies of cellular cytotoxic function has been extremely complex due to the existence of ubiquitous naturally-occurring cytotoxic cells (Heppner et al, 1975). Cytotoxicity should be measured only in selected well-controlled test populations, preferably by objective radiolabeled assays. We have used several radioactive markers in various projects and find that tritiated proline or Chromium-51 is suitable for labeling most target cells. Both methods may be used on a small scale in which only minimal numbers of reactive leukocytes and target cells are required. Selection of well-characterized target cells is also extremely important to any assay which purports to measure "specific" cytotoxicity in autoimmune disease or malignancy.

7. Macrophage Function

Because of the vital role of macrophages in the immune response, we are in the process of developing assays of such monocyte functions as chemotaxis and phagocytosis. The chemotactic response has been reported to be depressed in a number of disease states, including chronic and acute infections, malignancy, and diabetes (Territo and Cline, 1977). We are evaluating two methods for performing this assay, one which employs Chromium-51 labeled cells and another which evaluates chemotaxis by direct quantitation of stained monocytes. The phagocytic function may be decreased in immune deficiency syndromes and has been reported to be accelerated in cancer (Meltzer and Stevenson, 1978). The significance of these findings is unclear at the present time, but further investigation is warranted.

8. Summary

Methods in cellular immunology have developed to the point where they are accepted as an integral part of the clinical immunology laboratory, even though such methods are presently time-consuming and require technical expertise. Basic and applied immunological research, as well as laboratory application of semi-automatic techniques and careful quality control, can be expected to initiate changes in our approaches to measurement of cellular immunity.

The clinical laboratory has only recently acquired the basic knowledge and skills for analyses of cell reactivity. The contribution of cellular immunity assays to clinical pathology can be anticipated to become more meaningful as mechanisms of immunologic cell function become more clearly defined in health and disease.

9. References

Bloom, B. R. and David, J. R., eds. (1976). "In Vitro Methods in Cell-Mediated and Tumor Immunity," Academic Press, New York

Girard, J. P., Cattin, S. and Cuevas, M. (1976). *Ann Clin Res* **8**, 74-84

Heppner, G., Henry, E., Stolbach, L., Cummings, F., McDonough, E. and Calabresi, P. (1975). *Cancer Res* **35**, 1931-37

Levy, N. L., Auerbach, P. S. and Hayes, E. C. (1976). *N Engl J Med* **294**, 1423-27

Meltzer, M. S. and Stevenson, M. M. (1978). *Cell Immunol* **35**, 99-111

Rose, N. R. and Freedman, H., eds. (1976). "Manual of Clinical Immunology," American Society for Microbiology, Washington, D.C.

Territo, M. C. and Cline, M. J. (1977). *J Immunol* **118**, 187-92

Whiteside, T. L. and Rowlands, D. T. (1977). *Am J Path* **88**, 754-90

CHAPTER **II**

Future Trends and Applications of Cellular Immunity Procedures

T. YOSHIDA, M.D., D. Med. Sci.

Table of Contents

1. Introduction

It is extremely difficult, at the present time, for anyone to forsee future directions of cellular immunity procedures. This difficulty is apparent in view of at least 50 different experimental procedures which are currently available for the assessment of cellular immunity (reviewed in Bloom, 1971; David and David, 1972; Waksman, 1978). This consideration may justify my present approach for this topic, that is, to start discussion with some of the procedures used and examined closely in our own laboratory. It is my hope that proper analysis of these particular procedures may lead us to envision future trends and applications of cellular immunity procedures in general.

I would like to examine those procedures in two separate categories. First, I will discuss some procedures which have been in use for experimental animals although they have not yet been fully applied for clinical use. Then another set of experimental methods will be discussed; they are currently being developed in animal experiments and are expected to be useful in the future for clinical applications.

2. Applications of Available Procedures

A. Leukocyte Adherence Inhibition Assay (LAI)

This assay was initially developed by Halliday and his co-workers (1972; 1974). The assay is attractive since it needs minimum equipment, very few cells from peripheral blood, and takes a rather short time to complete. It was unclear, however, from original reports that the phenomenon actually reflects the delayed hypersensitivity state in animals. Therefore, we have started some basic studies on this procedure in guinea pigs (Yoshida, 1977), although initial studies were performed on men and mice.

Peripheral blood leukocytes are separated by sedimentation of red cells from 2-3ml of blood (the minimum may be 0.5-1.0ml) in 6% dextran solution. The leukocytes are washed in Hanks' balanced salt solution three times and resuspended in RPMI 1640 medium at cell concentration of 1×10^7/ml. Such cell suspension is put into small test tubes (12 $\times$ 75mm) with or without specific antigen, and incubated at 37°C for 30 minutes. After the incubation they are transferred onto a hemocytometer chamber and incubated for an additional period of 90 minutes. The number of cells on a given area of the chamber is counted before and after rinsing, and the percentage of adherent cells is calculated.

The indicator cells in this system were shown to be both lymphocytes and neutrophils rather than macrophages. Thus, peritoneal exudate cells from immune guinea pigs could not show LAI phenomenon when incubated with specific antigen. This is in contrast to macrophage migration inhibition phenomenon. Various evidences were obtained to indicate that the LAI is an in vitro correlate of delayed type hypersensitivity (DTH) (Yoshida, 1977): 1) A positive LAI was shown as early as five days after immunization with complete Freund's adjuvant (CFA) while no significant LAI was observed in guinea pigs immunized with incomplete Freund's adjuvant (IFA) throughout a six-week period following immunization. 2) The LAI is a carrier-specific phenomenon when hapten protein conjugates are used as antigens. 3) Antigen-antibody complex could not induce a positive LAI. 4) Cytophilic antibody could not mediate the LAI. 5) No difference was observed between leukocyte adherence in the medium with normal guinea pig serum and that in the medium with immune sera.

Does the LAI have any advantage as

an in vitro correlate of DTH conventional lymphokine assays—for example, macrophage migration inhibition (MMI) assay? As shown in Table I, the LAI needs less cells, less medium, and less time to complete one assay than the MMI. Furthermore, the LAI seems to be advantageous when humoral antibody of any sort is contaminated in the assay system since the assay is not affected by the presence of antigen-antibody complex. In this sense the LAI is a more specific phenomenon for the DTH than the MMI, since the MMI has been shown to be achieved by antigen-antibody complex as well as migration inhibition factor (MIF). Clinical applications of this assay have already started, especially on tumor immunity on an experimental scale (Halliday et al, 1974). As far as clinical applications are concerned, this procedure is suitable for the assessment of the DTH in pediatric patients from whom a rather small number of cells are available for any biological assays (Mukoyama et al, 1978).

B. Serum Lymphokine Activities—An Example of Cellular Immunity Mediators In Vivo

Although lymphokine production has been observed mainly in in vitro situations as described above, most lymphokines have been suggested as putative mediators of in vivo reactions of the cellular immunity based upon various indirect evidences (reviewed in Yoshida and Cohen, 1975; Yoshida et al, 1969). Direct evidence supporting this contention is scarce. About a decade ago, we showed that there was a prompt reduction in the number of circulating monocytes when rats or guinea pigs immunized with antigens in Freund's complete adjuvant were later challenged intravenously with large amounts of specific antigen (Yoshida et al, 1969). This effect of antigen on blood monocytes was a function of the state of delayed hypersensitivity of the animals.

Table I

COMPARISON BETWEEN LAI AND MMI

	LAI	MMI
Cell number[a]	$3-5 \times 10^5$	$3-5 \times 10^6$
Target Cells	Peripheral Leukocytes (lymphocytes and polymorphonuclear cells)	Peritoneal Exudates (macrophages or monocytes)
Antigen Concentration[b]	0.5 μg/ml	5 μg/ml
Medium[c]	0.1 ml	1.0 ml
Inhibition by Ag-Ab complex	No	Yes
Time necessary for assay	4-5 hours	24 hours

a. The minimal cell number necessary for testing a sample.

b. The least antigen concentration to be used for such antigen as DNP-BSA.

c. The minimal volume of culture medium necessary for a test.

Furthermore, we could detect MIF in the serum of such animals (Yoshida and Cohen, 1974). If one examines skin reactivity of these treated animals by specific antigen, delayed type skin reactions are found suppressed. This is a well-known phenomenon called the desensitization of delayed type hypersensitivity. Such detectability of MIF in the sera of desensitized animals has also been reported by several other laboratories in mice and guinea pigs (Yamamoto and Takehashi, 1971; Salvin et al, 1973).

More interestingly, the converse situation has also been studied (Yoshida and Cohen, 1974). Namely the in vitro generated lymphokines, including MIF, were injected intravenously into immunized guinea pigs. A control group of animals received the control culture supernatant. Following the administration of these materials, the animals were skin tested by specific antigen. As a result, 24-hour reactions were significantly reduced in intensity in the group of animals receiving the lymphokine-containing supernatant fluids. We were able to achieve a 50%-75% reduction in skin reaction size in these animals, as compared to those which had received the control supernatants.

These observations in experimental animals have clearly raised the possibility of detecting MIF activity in the sera of patients with various diseases. We chose to study the sera of patients with a variety of lymphoproliferative diseases, since lymphocytes from such patients may release MIF in culture in the absence of antigen challenge, and since those diseases are associated with alterations in immunologic status, which in some cases may be related to lymphokine-dependent mechanism. Out of 74 randomly chosen, putatively normal persons, only two serum samples have shown MIF-like activity. In contrast, a majority of the patients with lymphoproliferative diseases had MIF-like activity in their sera (Cohen et al, 1974). We obtained positive results in 14 of 16 patients with non-Hodgkin's lymphoma, 10 of 13 with Hodgkin's disease, and 4 of 5 with chronic lymphocytic leukemia. Two of three patients with myeloma showed activity. In another study of the lymphoproliferative diseases, the sera in all six cases of Sezary syndrome examined had MIF activity (Yoshida et al, 1975). In addition, the peripheral lymphocytes from some of these patients could produce MIF-like substance in vitro.

Along with those lymphoproliferative diseases, we have explored MIF activity in sera from patients with post-transplant hepatic disease (Torisu et al, 1973). MIF has been detected in the sera of six of eight patients with hepatic dysfunction following transplantation. None of the sera from five patients without hepatic dysfunction following transplantation had MIF activity. Serum MIF activity bore an interesting temporal relation to parameters of hepatic disease, especially serum glutamic oxaloacetic transaminase (SGOT) levels. Thus, elevations of serum MIF consistently preceded elevations of SGOT by approximately 5-10 days.

More recently, we have found that 26 (57%) of 46 patients with sarcoidosis exhibited serum MIF activity (Yoshida et al, 1978). Increased levels of MIF activity tended to be associated with a greater frequency of patient's failure to react to a battery of delayed-type hypersensitivity skin tests. These MIF activities in the sera of patients with the above mentioned diseases have been confirmed by various researchers (Bruley-Rosset et al, 1977; Umbert et al, 1976a; Umbert et al, 1976b). The clinical significance and implications of these observations, however, have yet to be exactly defined, although it is most likely that raised levels of MIF-like substance present in serum may be involved in the mechanism responsible for the relative anergy of patients with various diseases exemplified above.

C. General Trends

By discussing these two examples of procedures, I have attempted to indicate that apparently there would be two main directions in the development of cellular immunity procedures. One is exemplified by the LAI, that is, to search for a micro or even ultra-micro method which will require fewer numbers of cells and materials. In terms of the cell number necessary for an assay, the LAI was favorably considered over the MMI in the previous discussion. However, it should be noted that procedures have been developed to require fewer cells even in the MMI system. One such example is the agarose droplet method developed by Harrington and Stastny (1973). As another example, a lymphocyte transformation assay utilizing ^{3}H-thymidine uptake procedure has also been modified to achieve a convenient microsystem. Genius is not required to imagine a certain kind of single cell assay procedure towards the end of this trend. Theoretically, it is conceivable to develop single cell systems of, for instance, the MMI, chemotactic assays, blast transformation, macrophage activation, cytotoxic assays, and so on. Many laboratories seem to be working toward this direction.

The other trend of clinical applications in the future is exemplified by the detection of serum MIF in various experimental and clinical situations. Instead of using cells, one may only need to deal with soluble substances in this system. There are obvious and practical advantages in dealing with serum rather than live leukocytes or other cells obtained from a patient, as long as one can collect biologically or clinically relevant information. As mentioned above, the exact clinical significance of the serum MIF is not yet clear, and extensive studies must be carried out to determine if the MIF activity in serum does reflect a state of DTH in a given patient or not. If it does correlate with the DTH, however, the serum MIF assay would definitely give us a strong tool for the assessment of immunological competence of patients, as one can see in analogy to various mediator substances for immediate type hypersensitivity or various types of humoral antibodies. The serum MIF itself may turn out to be a minor or insignificant factor after all.

Nonetheless, several other lymphokines, lymphotoxins or chemotactic factors (Granger et al, 1978; Postlethwaite and Snyderman, 1974) in addition to MIF have already been reported in a variety of tissue fluids including serum, peritoneal or pleural cavity fluids, and joint fluids. Furthermore, factors which may regulate such lymphokines have also been reported in serum, for example, chemotactic factor inhibitors (Berenberg and Ward, 1973). In any event, what is essential here, and what I believe will be a future trend, is to obtain information on patient's capability of cellular immune responses by a cell-free procedure. Although the materials to be examined are cell-free, any known methods of detecting lymphokines at the present time still utilize cells from various sources as targets for their in vitro biological activities. Thus, the detection of serum MIF has obviated the use of cells from patients, but still needs to employ guinea pig macrophages for the assay. However, we may not need such target cells in the future since there is a strong possibility that a radioimmunoassay for lymphokines may be developed.

3. Future Development of New Procedures

In this section, I would like to discuss procedures which may be developed in the near future in experimental cellular immunity studies and hopefully applied to clinical immunology. Two newly developed procedures will be considered: one is a radioimmunoassay or equivalent procedure using anti-lymphokine serum, and the other is a procedure to generate effector cells in vitro, or to sensitize T-cells in vitro.

A. Immunofluorescence Studies and Radioimmunoassays of Lymphokines

It has been very difficult to produce antibody to the known lymphokines, because of a) the presence of lymphokines in minute quantities in activated lymphocyte culture supernatants and b) the presence of a large amount of contaminating materials in so-called "purified" preparations. Thus in the past, many attempts to produce antibody by immunizing animals with physicochemically purified lymphokines were unsuccessful, including our own experiences. In our laboratory, however, we have partially circumvented these difficulties by a two-stage immunization procedure (Yoshida et al, 1975).

Briefly, antiserum was raised against contaminating materials by immunizing rabbits with Sephadex G-100 column-fractionated control culture supernatants. This antiserum was termed anti-control serum. Lymphokine preparations partially purified by Sephadex G-100 gel filtration were then reacted with anti-control serum which was conjugated to agarose beads. Such immunoabsorption obviated the necessity for precipitating antibody in the system. By this means, we reduced the level of contaminants common to lymphokine and control preparations. Such immunochemically "purified" lymphokine preparations were then used as immunogen to obtain the final anti-lymphokine antiserum.

In spite of difficulties in raising anti-lymphokine antibody by a single stage procedure utilizing only physicochemically fractionated lymphokine preparation as immunogen, some investigators have reported success by such a direct approach. Thus, Geczy et al (1975) have obtained an anti-lymphokine serum by immunizing rabbits with lymphokine preparations prepared by physicochemical procedures including Sephadex G-200 and G-100 column chromatographies, Pevicon block electrophoresis, and polyacrylamide gel electrophoresis. Similarly, several laboratories have reported the production of anti-human lymphotoxin antisera (Walker and Lucas, 1974; Lewis et al, 1977; Hiserodt and Granger, 1977). All of these antisera have been found functionally able to neutralize lymphokine activities.

Nevertheless, any immunofluorescence or radioimmunoassays for lymphokines have yet to be seen utilizing these antisera. A major problem stems from the fact that currently available antisera are not yet pure enough to allow such procedures. One of the promising approaches has been described by Sorg and Geczy (1976). They have first labelled substances in the non-stimulated control lymphocyte cultured with ^{14}C-leucine, and cultures of the cells stimulated with antigen or mitogen are labeled with ^{3}H-leucine. By comparing the ratio of ^{3}H/^{14}C in fractions obtained

by the combined use of Sephadex G-75 gel filtration and isoelectric focusing on the labeled material, they could identify at least 14 products of activated lymphocytes synthesized either de novo or in increased amounts. Among them, at least five could bind specifically with anti-lymphokine antibody. Further studies would permit us to purify each of these materials and analyze the relationship among the molecules.

In any event, many laboratories are now engaged in one way or another obtaining a monospecific antibody if possible, or at least trying to obtain an antibody which is lymphokine-specific without any cross reactions with contaminants in lymphocyte culture supernatants. To achieve this, one can conceive various procedures: for example, a) vigorous physicochemical purification of the material obtained from immunoabsorption procedures, b) vigorous absorption of antisera with possible contaminants, or c) immunize animals with immunochemically partially "purified" lymphokines to obtain a second stage antiserum.

Once we obtain an antiserum which is satisfactorily usable for immunofluorescence and/or radioimmunoassays, the current state of the art in the latter procedures would permit us to study precisely the in vivo significance of lymphokines as discussed in the previous section and eventually to understand physiology and pathology of mediator production in cell-mediated immunity.

B. Induction of Cellular Immunity In Vitro

It may be evident that the discussion up to this point has been concerned with only the effector phase of cellular immunity. This is mainly because we know virtually nothing about the induction phase of this type of immune response. In antibody response, on the other hand, we have a fairly good understanding of the initial phase of its production, and conveniently, there are various in vitro antibody production systems available, permitting us to analyze the actual event taking place in lymphoid organs. Thus, primary antibody production system in vitro is already clinically in use to assess the ability of various lymphocyte populations from patients.

In the field of cellular immunity, the only procedure available for primary induction of effector cells in vitro is the induction of cytotoxic T-cells by either mixed leukocyte cultures or mixed leukocyte-tumor cell cultures (Bloom and David, 1976). Cytotoxicity mediated by T-lymphocytes is a very important aspect, but definitely not a general mechanism of cellular immunity. It would be a tremendous advantage to have an in vitro system to generate lymphocytes capable of producing lymphokines. Based on our knowledge of necessary conditions to generate antibody-forming cells in vitro or cytotoxic T-cells from either spleens or lymph nodes, the time is ripe for an attempt to establish a method generating lymphokine-producing cells (or mediator cells for delayed type hypersensitivity) in vitro. Establishment of such procedures will make it possible for us to analyze the developmental process of antigen sensitive T-cells, probably the requirement of accessory cells, various cellular interactions, a critical stage of lymphocyte differentiation which may separate it from the antibody-forming process, etc. Consequently, our understanding of patho-physiology in the induction phase of cell-mediated immunity in human will be facilitated.

C. General Comments

A large number of novel techniques in the field of cellular immunity and their application to human disease have been developed especially during the last decade (Bloom and David, 1976; Rose and Friedman, 1976). We may expect similar rapid evolution of newer

and better techniques and procedures to continue for some time. Naturally, it is beyond the scope of this article to consider future trends in every conceivable aspect of experimental cellular immunity procedures. By discussing only two aspects of evolving procedures in cellular immunity, I have attempted to predict the central trend in the development of procedures in the future. This predicted trend, together with currently available procedures, is summarized in Figure 1 (next page) and somewhat extended to general comments described below.

One of the most likely and desirable trends in the future of this field is to develop a cell-free in vitro procedure. In almost all of the cellular immunity procedures, the critical problem has been technical difficulties in controlling and standardizing (if not uncontrollable) various parameters associated with living target cells used for in vitro assays. This has been the main reason that most of the currently available assays for cellular immunity are, at best, qualitative without permitting us any quantitative analysis of data. Fortunately, the possibility seems to be strong that a cell-free method may be developed for in vitro assays of cellular immunity, especially for the detection of lymphokines.

Nevertheless, there is still a possibility that the use of live cells remains an absolute requirement for some assays. For these, it may become important to standardize the cells to be used as much as possible. An essential development is the use of established cell lines or at least well-characterized homogeneous cells rather than the use of primary cultured cells such as peritoneal exudate cells. In this respect, encouraging attempts have already begun in the use of established macrophage cell lines, or creation of useful target and/or effector cells by cell-hybridization techniques (Bloom, 1978).

Furthermore, in an extension of this

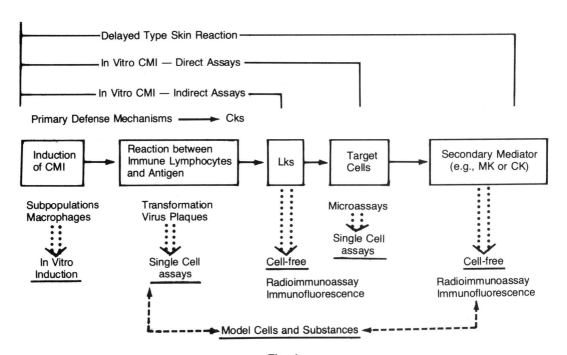

Fig. 1

FUTURE TREND IN CELL-MEDIATED IMMUNITY (CMI) PROCEDURES

Stages of CMI responses are shown in blocks □. Examples of possible future development in procedures are indicated by broken lines and arrows, while currently available three groups of CMI procedures are shown in the upper section of this figure.

trend, we can see probably development of an "artificial" model system for the studies on cellular immunity. This can be considered at two different levels: a model for the cell and models for mediators. For example, in some cellular immune assay procedures, it may be conceivable to substitute the target cell with a certain type of artificial (or model) membrane. In fact, phospholipid bilayers in vesicular form (liposomes) have been successfully utilized as substrates for immune attack by complement (Kinsky, 1972; Kinsky et al, 1969). The possibility that liposomes might serve as target membranes for cell-mediated cytotoxic attack has been explored by Ozato et al (1978), although initial attempts have encountered various technical difficulties.

As to model molecules for mediators, several tripeptides have been shown to possess strong chemotactic activity for neutrophils (Showell et al, 1976). Although it is unknown at the present time if other lymphokine activities can also be mimicked by these simple peptides, such simple molecules used in combinations with the above-mentioned membranes could give us a tool to construct a model system to study the complex events between lymphokines and target cells. This would eventually make it feasible to examine the activities of physiological factors (e.g. lymphokines and inflammatory cells) by simply introducing the material to be tested into the model system.

Another major trend for cellular immunity procedures is the invention of a method for studying its induction mechanism. The rapid development of such procedures is urgent since virtually no practical method is available in contrast to the many procedures described for effector cells and substances in cellular immunity.

4. Concluding Remarks

Future trends and applications of cellular immunity procedures discussed above are obviously based upon my own biased grasp of the current state of the art in this field. Naturally, we must wait for some time to see if any of these predictions may come true. As a summary of this small article, however, let me daydream further and try to visualize a picture of a clinical laboratory where various tests are performed to evaluate the cellular immune reactivity of a given patient one day in the near future.

A small volume of blood or other tissue fluids is obtained. Cellular and humoral components are automatically separated by centrifugation, and humoral components are analyzed for concentrations of various lymphokine molecules and their inhibitors or regulators. Any abnormality of these contents in a sample is easily noticed in comparison with normal values. Cellular components are first labeled by immunofluorescence or radioactive materials according to their cell surface or intracellular antigens, and then separated into different populations by a cell-sorter which has the ability to separate the cells according to the combined characteristics of sizes, fluorescent properties, and radioactivity. The distribution pattern of the patient's cells in each fraction makes it easy for one to realize any abnormal cellular profile at a glance. Several cells from each fraction are then mixed in a desired fashion and cultured in an appropriate manner to observe their functional abilities, including the ability to generate cytotoxic cells and antigen-primed T-cells, the ability to react as target cells for chemotaxis, phagocytosis, and the ability to produce lymphokines.

In any event, regardless of actual procedures used in the future, I am certain that laboratory data obtained from cellular immunity procedures will become more essential in the diagnosis and prognosis of disease, as it is the vehicle for many important clinical assays such as, for example, determination of blood sugars, enzymes, or urea, and detection of malignant cells or abnormal erythrocytes.

5. References

Berenberg, J. L. and Ward, P. A. (1973). *J Clin Invest* **52**, 1200

Bloom, B. R. (1971). *Adv Immunol* **13**, 101

Bloom, B. R. (1978). *Fed Proc* In press

Bloom, B. R. and David, J. R., eds. (1976). "In Vitro Methods in Cell-Mediated and Tumor Immunity," Academic Press, New York

Bruley-Rosset, M., Botto, H. G. and Goutner, A. (1977). *Eur J Cancer* **13**, 325

Cohen, S., Fisher, B., Yoshida, T. and Bettigole, R. (1974). *N Eng J Med* **290**, 882

David, J. R. and David, R. A. (1972). *Prog Allergy* **16**, 300

Geczy, C. L., Friedrich, W. and de Weck, A. L. (1975). *Cell Immunol* **19**, 65

Granger, G. A., Shimizer, I., Harris, L., Anderson, J. and Horn, P. (1978). *Clin Immunol Immunopathol* **10**, 104

Halliday, W. J., Maluish, A. E. and Ispister, W. H. (1974). *Br J Cancer* **29**, 31

Halliday, W. J. and Miller, S. (1972). *Int J Cancer* **9**, 477

Harrington, J. T. and Stastny, P. (1973). *J Immunol* **110**, 752

Hiserodt, J. C. and Granger, G. A. (1977). *J Immunol* **119**, 374

Kinsky, S. C. (1972). *Biochem Biophys Acta* **265**, 1

Kinsky, S. C., Haxby, J. A., Zopt, D. A., Alving, C. R. and Kinsky, C. B. (1969). *Biochem* **8**, 4149

Lewis, J. E., Carmack, C. E., Yamamoto, R. and Granger, G. A. (1977). *J Immunol Meth* **14**, 163

Mukoyama, T., Kuratsuji, T. and Yoshida, T. (1978). *Jap J Allerg* **27**, 393

Ozato, K., Ziegler, K. and Henney, C. S. (1978) *J Immunol* **121**, 1383

Postlethwaite, A. E. and Snyderman, R. (1974). *J Immunol* **114**, 274

Rose, N. R. and Friedman, H., eds. (1976). "Manual of Clinical Immunology," American Society of Microbiology, Washington, D.C.

Salvin, S. B., Youngner, J. S. and Lederer, W. H. (1973). *Infect Immun* **7**, 68

Showell, H. J., Freer, R. J., Zigmond, S. H., Schiffmann, E., Aswadumar, S., Corcoran, B. and Becker, E. L. (1976). *J Exp Med* **143**, 1154

Sorg, C. and Geczy, C. L. (1976). *Europ J Immunol* **6**, 688

Torisu, M., Yoshida, T., Ward, P. A. and Cohen, S. (1973). *J Immunol* **111**, 1450

Umbert, P., Belcher, R. W. and Winkelmann, R. K. (1976a). *Brit J Dermatol* **95**, 475

Umbert, P., Belcher, R. W. and Winkelmann, R. K. (1976b). *Brit J Dermatol* **95**, 481

Waksman, B. H. (1978). *Pharmacol Review* In press

Walker, S. M. and Lucas, Z. J. (1974). *J Immunol* **113**, 813

Yamamoto, K. and Takahashi, Y. (1971). *Nature* **233**, 261

Yoshida, T. (1977). *In* "Regulatory Mechanisms in Lymphocyte Activation" (Lucas, D., ed.) p. 665, Academic Press, New York

Yoshida, T. and Cohen, S. (1974). *J Immunol* **112**, 1540

Yoshida, T. and Cohen, S. (1974). *In* "Mechanisms of Cell-Mediated Immunity" (McCluskey, R. T. and Cohen, S., eds.) p. 43, J. Wiley & Sons, New York

Yoshida, T. and Cohen, S. (1975). *In* "The Immune System and Infectious Diseases" (Neter, E. and Milgrom, F., eds.) p. 512, Karger, Basel, Switzerland

Yoshida, T., Benacerraf, B., McCluskey, R. T. and Vassalli, P. (1969). *J Immunol* **102**, 804

Yoshida, T., Bigazzi, P. E. and Cohen, S. (1975). *J Immunol* **114**, 688

Yoshida, T., Edelson, R., Cohen, S. and Green, I. (1975). *J Immunol* **114**, 915

Yoshida, T., Siltzbach, L. E. and Cohen, S. (1978). VIIIth International Congress of Sarcoidosis, Cardiff, Wales

CHAPTER III

Quality Control and Standards for Cellular Immunology

N. R. ROSE, M.D., Ph.D.

Table of Contents

1. Introduction

The field of cellular immunology is the newest and most rapidly growing facet of clinical immunology. Consequently, methods of quality control are still nascent and standards virtually non-existent.

The subject will be discussed at two levels: general problems of quality control and specific considerations related to individual test procedures.

2. General Considerations

The general principles of quality control pertinent to other areas of laboratory medicine are applicable generally to the study of human cellular immunological functions. They include the parameters of sensitivity, specificity, clinical accuracy, clinical relevance, and determination of normal range.

As applied to cellular immunology, sensitivity implies the lower limit of detection of an immunological response. In general, cellular immunological reactions have a high degree of sensitivity, often extending beyond the range of clinical usefulness. Specificity describes the ability of the reaction to distinguish between antigens, that is, the responsiveness of a patient or a patient's cells to one antigen and not to other unrelated or only distantly related antigens. As in all immunological reactions, specificity is relative, and in high ranges of sensitivity, specificity is diminished. Many naturally occurring molecules share individual antigenic determinants, and, if a sufficiently sensitive test procedure is employed, cross-reactions can be expected. In addition, one sometimes encounters fortuitous cross-reactions due to identical antigenic determinants found on two different biological molecules, that is, heterogenetic or heterophilic reactions. While better known in humoral immunology, similar unexpected cross-reactions can be encountered in cellular immunological assays.

Clinical accuracy denotes the ability of a test to detect all cases of a particular abnormality or disease and none other. Obviously, such a parameter must be based on the accuracy of clinical diagnosis, which itself is a subjectively determined variable. Nevertheless, sensitivity and specificity of immunological reactions must be interpreted on a clinical scale.

One frequently sees the term "false positive" in the literature, implying that a reaction occurs in instances where the physician does not expect it. These reactions may be technical failures or may exemplify the occurrence of an immunological response in instances other than the disease under consideration. The term "biological false positive" is often applied to this latter category. The term is an unfortunate one, because there is nothing false about the reaction in these instances. It is a perfectly correct observation, although it does not coincide with our predetermined clinical diagnosis. It is based on the fact that immunological responses can occur due to a variety of stimuli and not just to a single stimulus.

The term "false negative" is often used in a similar vein, indicating the lack of an expected immunological response in patients with a particular clinical diagnosis. The failure may be due to limited technical sensitivity of the method or due to the fact that the particular patient failed to develop an expected immunological response. Here again there is nothing false about these negatives, and they may provide useful insight into the spectrum of responses underlying immunological disorders.

The performance of tests for cellular immunological functions is generally time-consuming and expensive. Our understanding of their importance in the diagnosis and treatment of disease is still at a relatively primitive stage. Therefore, many measurements that are technically possible in the laboratory add little to our knowledge of the clinical situation. In the case of cellular immunological reactions, one often finds derangements that are secondary or tertiary consequences of the underlying derangement. Moreover, they may not represent a level of impairment that is reflected in clinical susceptibility. This situation arises because of the great sensitivity of immunological measures described above. It is often possible to detect changes in immunological function that seem to have very little influence on the course or outcome of disease. While it may be of great interest and future importance to demonstrate these subtle changes in order to increase our understanding of immunological responses, their measurement cannot presently be justified as a regular clinical procedure. It is more sensible to carry out such tests in the context of an investigation where all of the necessary data can be collected and analyzed in order to add to the store of immunological knowledge.

Finally, very few cellular immunological tests are "all or none." In most cases, patients show some response which may be magnified or diminished in disease. It is the degree of change that must be determined. Often this requires repeated measurements in the same individual. Moreover, these functions differ with age, sex, racial group, environmental exposure, and many other details of past history. It is often difficult or impossible to determine whether a value is normal or abnormal without possessing considerable knowledge about the past and present history of the particular patient under consideration. Therefore, tests of cellular immunity are rarely interpretable as "blind" determinations. They usually require close interaction between the laboratorian and clinician to arrive at an intelligent interpretation.

Because of their complexity, assays of cell-mediated immunity are rarely as accurate or precise as other clinical laboratory procedures. To reduce variability, careful attention is necessary to all details of the test. A high level of technical ability is required. Unfortunately, it is rarely possible to repeat determinations of samples taken from the same patient over a period of time, as is customary in humoral immunology. Therefore, it is often difficult to know whether an abnormal value represents a real biological change or a technical variation. For this reason, repeated assays are often required. Whenever possible, more than one type of test should be performed in order to give complementary information. Added confidence results from tests that independently reveal the same type of abnormality, while an individual abnormal finding is, by itself, rarely diagnostic.

3. Specific Test Procedures

Generally, the most useful single test for the assessment of cell-mediated immunity is the delayed hypersensitivity skin test performed upon the patient himself. The accuracy of this test depends upon the quality of the skin test reagent, and the skill with which it is applied and read by the physician. Some skin test antigens, such as PPD or SK/SD, are rather well characterized and can be purchased in standard units. Other reagents, such as Candida antigen (dermatophyton) or tricophyton, are sold merely as dilutions of a company's standard preparation. In these cases, it is important to purchase the material from a vendor of good repute.

The correct administration and scoring of the test are often neglected or left to untrained personnel. Erroneous results frequently ensue. It is important that the physician understand that an interdermal skin test must be truly interdermal, that the reaction be read properly for induration, and that repeated readings be recorded over a 72-hour period so that delayed hypersensitivity can be distinguished from other types of hypersensitivity responses. It is also important to remember that a negative reaction may result from the inability of the patient to mobilize lymphocytes and/or macrophages. For example, treatment with steroid hormones may lead to negative responses in otherwise responsive patients with underlying cell-mediated immunity.

In vitro measures of cell-mediated immunity are becoming increasingly common. They should begin with a careful assessment of total leukocyte populations, including morphological study of a differential blood film. The relative and absolute numbers of T- and B-cells can now be determined with reasonable accuracy in most individuals. T-cell enumeration usually depends upon E-rosette formation, although antisera to T-cells and subsets of T-cells are rapidly becoming available. Several assays for B-cells are available, including surface immunoglobulin markers, Fc receptors, and complement receptors. All of these tests require biological reagents that are often variable. For example, the source of sheep red blood cells influences the number of E-rosetting lymphocytes. Therefore, it is essential that each reagent be carefully studied in advance or obtained from an established investigator.

Null cell determinations are usually made by subtraction. It is possible to subcategorize null cells by in vitro cultivation in the presence or absence of thymic hormone. Again, these procedures are quite variable from laboratory to laboratory.

In addition to determination of T- and B-cell numbers in peripheral blood, it is possible to perform lymphocyte quantitation on tissues. These methods may be particularly helpful in cases of lymphoproliferative malignancy. However,

when dealing with abnormal lymphocytes either from peripheral blood or tissues, the immunologist must recognize that he is likely to obtain aberrant results. Often these problems can be solved only by referring the specimen or the patient to a center with greater experience in this sort of determination.

For in vitro cultivation, cells of peripheral blood are usually taken from a heparinized sample. Sometimes lymphoid organs, such as tonsils or spleen, are used. It is important that lymphocytes be separated from other blood and tissue elements as quickly as possible, preferably within a few hours of drawing. Once separated, it is possible to store lymphocytes overnight in the refrigerator with little evidence of change in their activity.

Methods of cultivation and assay differ greatly from laboratory to laboratory. It is rarely possible to relate findings in one center to another. Therefore, it is important that each laboratory establish the normal range expected for individuals of various ages.

For detection of migration inhibitory factor, either direct or indirect methods may be used. The indirect test using guinea pig peritoneal exudate cells generally seems to be more reproducible, but technically more demanding. It is likely that the direct tests using the patient's own monocytes as indicators actually measure a different lymphokine function. Although a few centers are capable of carrying out tests for other lymphokines, such as interferon, lymphotoxin, or lymphocyte mitogenic factor, most clinical laboratories will find these procedures beyond their capabilities.

Methods for determining chemotaxis and phagocytosis are necessary in order to evaluate most cases of untoward susceptibility to infection. Some of the methods, such as ingestion of opsonized particles, are relatively simple to perform as long as one realizes that they depend upon living cells. Therefore, it is important that proper care be given to taking and separating the phagocytic cells from the blood specimen, that glassware be properly free of toxic reagents, that temperature and nutrients be properly controlled, and that the tests be done promptly enough so that cell injury does not interfere. While tests of chemotaxis and phagocytosis are applicable to macrophages as well as polymorphonuclear phagocytes, they are much less commonly done because of the difficulty of finding sufficient numbers of well-functioning monocytes in peripheral blood.

4. Summary

At present, the best test of cellular immunity is still the delayed hypersensitivity skin test. Reasonable well-characterized and standardized reagents are available, and, if proper care is exercised in their application and reading, acceptable results can be expected. In vitro tests of cell-mediated immunity are still in a developmental stage. Almost all clinical immunological laboratories can now carry out enumeration of T- and B-lymphocytes with considerable precision, although results may differ from laboratory to laboratory. Lymphocyte proliferative responses and the elaboration of lymphokine are more variable, but usually can be performed in a satisfactory manner.

The simpler tests of chemotaxis and phagocytosis are also widely applicable. On the other hand, many other biological assay systems are still in a stage where they are best performed only in larger investigative centers, where sufficient experience can be accumulated in carrying out the tests and interpreting the results.

Part I

DISCUSSION PERIOD

DR. RITZMANN: It seems that we in the immunodiagnostic laboratories are faced with the same dilemma which pharmacologists solved decades ago when they abandoned the practice of individually preparing their own therapeutic formulations and started to depend upon quality controlled, commercially available drugs. Today, with the ever-increasing availability of diagnostic kits and preparations, we are entering a similar phase, allowing us to avoid "re-inventing the wheel" in our individual laboratories and hopefully to also contribute to the cost containment of diagnostic measures. Therefore, the various viewpoints presented and discussed this morning are of considerable relevance, providing a basis for a general agreement on our requirements for the various immunodiagnostic areas and procedures, including quality standards for commercial preparations.

DR. HURTUBISE: We had the opportunity about two years ago to study a selected panel of patient's sera with increased bilirubin content, lipemia, immune complexes, and monoclonal immunoglobulins of various light and heavy chain specificity.

This study was done in collaboration with Dr. Neil Davis at the Children's Hospital in Cincinnati, Ohio. Serum immunoglobulins (IgG, IgA, and IgM) on these 150 patient samples were quantitated by immunodiffusion, nephelometric light-scattering, and fluorometric methods. The instruments employed included the Hyland nephelometer, the Beckman rate analyzer, the Behring nephelometer, the Kallestad nephelometer, the Technicon automated immunoprecipitin system, and the fluorometric IDT and BioRad systems. Each of the manufacturers supplied the reagents and the instruments used. Linear regression analyses between the various methods for quantitating immunoglobulins consistently showed a correlation coefficient of approximately 0.7. The greatest disparity was observed when sera obtained from myeloma patients were studied. There was also some bias in icteric specimens when assayed by the fluorometric methods.

The specimens were processed as routine specimens by the medical technologists in the laboratory. We found that the biggest problem in the various commercial assays involved the absence of an accurate serum dilution system, which is probably responsible for significant variations in assay results. We feel the problem with some assays is not instrumentation, but reagent control at the manufacturer's level.

For example, in the study of a patient with IgA immunodeficiency disease, two of the instrument systems had assay values of 120ng per 100ml of IgA, while other instrument systems were reporting zero. The patient truly did have an IgA deficiency. The discrepancy was related to one manufacturer's use of goat antisera versus another's use of rabbit antisera. The falsely elevated value of IgA was caused by the presence of anti-goat antibodies in the IgA deficient patient. Hence, major problems are related to standardization of reagents.

DR. RITCHIE: The problem with IgA determinations is easily solved. The process is simply that bovine or caprine IgM must be removed from the antisera since this is the antigen to which IgA deficient individuals produce precipitating antibody.

DR. HORAN: Has the Milstein technique for the production of specific antisera been used by some members of this group? It is clear that this is the method of choice for making antibodies. The Milstein technique involves the use of mice, hyperimmunized to a specific antigen, and three days after the last boost, the spleen is removed. Isolated spleen cells are then fused with a non-immunoglobulin producing myeloma cell such as the X63NS type. The spleen and continuous myeloma cells are fused with polyethylene glycol. The hybrid cells are selected in HAT media and then cloned in tissue cultures. As a result, individual clones producing antibodies according to the direction of the mouse B- cell are isolated and recultured. The desired clone will produce a monoclonal antibody. These cell lines can be frozen and stored in a viable state to be recultured as needed to produce mouse anti-IgG, anti-IgE, etc. It would be interesting to make the comparison between antibodies produced by animals vs. hybridoma methods employing a nephelometric technique or an absorption technique. Each time an antisera is produced from the animals, the animal responds to a different set of antigenic determinants on the specific antigen. With the mouse myeloma system, standard uniform monoclonal antibody can be maintained indefinitely.

DR. RITCHIE: It is extremely important that this has been mentioned. We recognize the fact that gearing up to produce antisera in thousands of liters by an in vitro technique is some years away. We know that antisera produced against an individual purified protein in animals have many reactivities and are not specifically reactive against one portion of a given molecule. However, the in vitro monoclonal antibody will have limited antigenic reactivity to a complex protein molecule.

DR. CAWLEY: There is some utility in noticing that the patient does have antibodies against goat or other species such as guinea pig. One technique which provides this capability is immunoelectrophoresis; when accurately performed, this technique will detect extra bands against other species. Immunoelectrophoresis is a very convenient back-up, preventing errors with gel diffusion and nephelometry as well.

DR. NAKAMURA: The hybridoma technique for in vitro antibody production is not far into the future. Antihormone antibodies with very high titers can be produced. The cloning of the desired antibody and specificity may be very difficult.

We need to discuss the production of a standard for gel and nephelometric methods.

DR. KEITGES: It is our plan to produce a calibrator or standard which will be made available to the proficiency testing survey through the CAP. Dr. Nakamura and I conferred with Dr. Reimer at the CDC. It was Dr. Reimer's suggestion that we use glass vials with siliconized tops containing a standard very similar to CDC candidate preparation number 3. However, the reference value is now in question. As Dr. Ritzmann pointed out, we can rely on the manufacturer, who obviously would individually enjoy having his standard accepted as the class standard.

DR. NAKAMURA: At that point in time, Dr. Reimer felt that we should seek a reputable person to begin production of 20mg of the purified antigen for the primary standard. Clinically, we wanted standards for immunoglobulins C_3 and C_4; it is felt the production of standards for the five proteins would be a real achievement. The availability of purified antigens for those five proteins would enable us to supply purified antigens to various laboratories. At this time, I would like to poll the opinion of the group.

DR. KEITGES: This plan has the blessings of the group from the IUIS and Dr. Reimer.

Again, the goal is to develop a secondary standard which would be immediately referable to CDC candidate number 3, and was part of the paper which Dr. Reimer planned to present. The College has sent out production specifications in order that bids might be generated by some of the manufacturers.

DR. NAKAMURA: The Hyland Company had the contract for the standards of the College. Discussion was held with the Hyland Group and Calbiochem-Behring. However, Dr. Ritchie has a standard that is very good; if we can accept the primary values and come to some consensus, we might arrive at a point of reference.

DR. KEITGES: This ad hoc committee was challenged to develop a standard for the World Health Organization through the International Union on Immunological Societies. Thus, candidate preparation number 3 was prepared at the CDC. The information regarding the need for the production of the secondary standard will be published very soon. It was felt that there was no method of correlating the CAP proficiency testing with manufacturer's standards. All manufacturers are producing good material, but there is a need to compare one with another. It is our aim to develop this secondary standard which is referable to the primary standard; the College would then send this standard to the participant. In addition to providing material to test for immunoglobulins common, the participant would have the secondary standard. The number of laboratories in the CAP proficiency is well over 2000 and we could now include them in that particular phase of proficiency testing. There are about 12,000 labs in the program. Baseline could then be established. Offering this standard to the laboratory at large is another consideration.

We are continually impressed with the tremendous value of exposing the materials used in the CAP proficiency testing program. The immediate possibility of having the material sent to thousands of laboratories is an extremely valuable tool for some of the testing. Bob, Dr. Reimer, and I are very excited about this possibility. Any statements regarding this very real possibility or some pitfalls to be avoided would be graciously received. Viewing the specifications for this material indicates that it may be very expensive. We are now awaiting the bids of industry for the cost of production.

DR. HURTUBISE: In connection with the proposed standard, I recommend the development of a high standard as well as a low standard.

I have a question which I would like to address to the speakers this morning. Does the nature of molecules influence, to some degree, how they perform in a nephelometric analysis, for example, IgM?

DR. RITCHIE: Yes, indeed they do. Glycoproteins are difficult to use, and the curves that Dr. Lawrence Killingsworth showed for orosomucoid are characteristic of that very problem. The source of the protein also makes a difference. This is why Dr. Reimer has stressed parallelism studies for preparations to show whether they are, in fact, similar to standard materials before they are accepted as a Standard. In the past, arbitrary units have been assigned to protein standards; for example, the International Units were attached to the Immunoglobulin Standard. Many people are upset by the lack of an absolute gravimetric unit. Does it make a difference to clinical medicine to have an absolute number which is biochemically proper?

On a practical basis, even albumin quantitation in absolute gravimetric units is subject to a great deal of difficulty in this regard. If this problem with albumin exists, one can certainly appreciate the problems with quantitative expression of C_3 or proteins less stable than C_3. This problem was again exemplified by a conference last May at the N.I.H. on the subject of alpha-feto protein (AFP). Many desired a purified AFP standard. While it may be quite practical to produce a vial which contains "X" mg of the purified material, is it immunologically identical? The analytical goal should be based on clinical relevance and not necessarily accuracy and precision alone as an end in itself. In other words, the immunopotency of a purified standard needs to be documented. What has happened to it during the process of purification? How does it react during a test? I'll cite you an example of this problem. Purified transferrin can be easily made in large quantities. One mg of purified transferrin per ml may be assayed by a mass technique, and when serum is added to it, a recovery of half the mass value may be obtained by standard immunoclinical assays. Something happens to it in the purified state when taken away from its native environment. This phenomenon has been well documented in enzymology. It may be advisable to consider laboratory experiments and clinical relevance rather than to expend all our energies in the quest of accurate mass units of questionable biological behavior. The performance of the laboratory may be the ultimate measuring instrument.

DR. NAKANE: In terms of the future, in any system where the essential prerequisite is formation of a precipitate using immunologic specificity as a criteria for the assay, we will come to narrowing of antigenic determinant specificity and to a point where the antibody will become monoclonal. I predict, therefore, that in the majority of instances where antigen is measured, a precipitate will not be formed.

In such circumstances, I can see one or two other ways of making an artificial multi-antigenic compound competing with the natural unknown substance, etc. What are the current thoughts of the future of a particular system, then, that requires precipitation as a prerequisite, but in which one will not expect a precipitate to form?

DR. SAVORY: I would hesitate to comment too much. Referring to precipitates, they perhaps are not precipitates, but large particles in the form of a pseudo-colloidal suspension. I just want to completely disagree with Bob Ritchie's statements about accuracy and precision. We ought to divide up the problem into two sections: (1) Try to produce good results, and (2) Answer your question, "So what?" This will present a real problem. At the Clinical Chemistry Aspen Conference two years ago, there was acceptance of a recommendation in clinical chemistry that we were dealing in numbers. That is, the precision of the assay should be about one-third the intra-individual variation of the test. That is not a bad rule of thumb. In proteins of the intra-individual variation, it's very, very low. Dr. Lawrence Killingsworth showed, very nicely, real consistency of all these protein assays, one or two percent over a matter of a week, and it is probably over a matter of years as well. I've been in a recent situation where the clinical laboratory has been in a real mess. None of the tests were precise, none of the tests were accurate, and the laboratory was a real mess. I think we're going to cause confusion if we say, "Well, this precision is satisfactory for this protein, 30% is satisfactory, 50% is satisfactory." Let's work with accurate and precise methods and then address the problem of the clinical utility. I believe a group such as this can address that problem. Let's try to pick the proteins which might be important and see how they really fit into the clinical setting. Are the acute phase proteins important to clinical medicine? Is a profile of this type important? If we can address that problem separately from the accuracy and precision, we'll really be accomplishing something.

DR. CHANDOR: I feel that it is important to reemphasize that in running the clinical immunology lab, regardless of hospital size, one frequently must deal with clinicians. The clinician will react to the kind of results we're going to produce. One of the aspects Dr. Ritchie brought up is the variation of a population to produce a "normal range." Meloy brought this out with their national study. Maybe it is part of the committee's function to emphasize this variation of a given area—population—and not to completely rely on what has been given out by a committee or a company as to the "normal range" of a test result, such as a protein level. Another area is the monoclonal proteins. If just one of the three types of evaluations is done, whether it is quantitation, electrophoresis, or immunoelectrophoresis, on occasion a monoclonal protein has been missed or incorrectly classified. Perhaps the committee should suggest that if one is going to evaluate monoclonal proteins, that one have the capabilities for doing more than one of the evaluation techniques.

DR. RITZMANN: Just an amplifying statement about monoclonal gamopathies. Regarding the standardization of the various assay procedures for immunoglobulins, as well as other proteins, consideration should be given to the assay ranges offered by these methods. For instance, several commercial RID plates either do not cover what we consider to be the normal protein ranges, or extend to extremely high, but irrelevant, levels at the exclusion of the clinically relevant assay ranges.

DR. KEITGES: Dr. Nakamura and I would like either on a collective or individual basis to get a feeling from the conference about what they really think is necessary to develop a definitive purified equation on this primary material, or simply for the sake of this secondary standard to establish a baseline and the World Health Organization could assign values to it and just proceed from there as if that were home plate. Any comments from the audience?

DR. HURTUBISE: I think you have to define the problem. What are you measuring? Are you measuring 1, 2, 3 and 4 subclasses? Does variability of subclasses in patients give you differences? When you define the standard, is it necessary to go back to the base definition? The same thing is true with IgA, and if that can be defined adequately, and it must be defined clinically, its development must be such that there is clinical relevance in the definition process. I agree that there should be a standard, but there are many questions underlining that standard.

DR. KEITGES: If we ever reached a point at any time, during any discussion period, where the group felt strongly about something, the Conference could adopt a resolution such as the one in clinical chemistry—that precision is defined roughly, and this is a useful definition. Friday we will try to summate each discussion group's deliberations. We will then get the Conference to convert these to resolution or proposal form at that point, so that the proceedings will have some definitive steps of improvement included in them.

DR. RITZMANN: Obviously, numerous problems remain to be solved, and the ongoing discussions should aid us in the formulation of the appropriate proposals by the end of this meeting.

Part II

DISCUSSION PERIOD

DR. TENOSO: After Dr. Ritchie's comment this morning of "so what," I became guilt-ridden about what my role would be here. The guilt centered around whether my presence would eventually contribute to improved health care or merely to its increased cost. To examine what we've heard today in a different light, I'll throw out a few numbers that may or may not prove helpful.

There are approximately five billion tests of a clinical nature run in the U.S. during the course of one year. (These are 1976-77 figures.) Of these, the immunoassay market, and that is what we are talking about, amounts to about $100 million in terms of total dollar volume. There are only six tests which comprise about 80% of this market. They include the thyroid assays, the T3 and T4 uptake in terms of hormone assays, and hepatitis in infectious disease testing. CEA tests make up a very large portion of cancer tests. In the drug tests, the largest volume test is the digoxin assay, and there are a number of other tests coming along. Just in terms of total volume of tests run today, digoxin is probably by far the greatest. Rubella tests comprise a significant part of the total volume of the immunoassays.

All of these tests cover the major portion of the immunoassay testing in terms of dollars. Of this group, about 80% is RIA, and it is the RIA group where the potential probably lies for EIA. The replacement will certainly not happen overnight or even over the next five or ten years. As Dr. Walls mentioned, the creation of standards is a laborious process. One of the traps we encounter is that we create a standard for a test today that isn't needed when it becomes available.

According to Dr. Nakane, some of the things we talked about today might not be applicable in terms of standards in the next five to ten years. So one of the considerations is that the standard, or at least the criteria, should be adjustable for the new techniques and, if possible, be applicable for five years. But there are several problems. The manufacturer would like guidelines for standards. We are concerned with quality and that various laboratories get the same results. The people on the advisory committees to FDA regulatory agencies also need some kind of information as to what their criteria should be, and of course, so does the individual laboratory. And last, but not least, is that with the advent of some of these tests, e.g. EIA for rubella antibody, you have this other dilemma now of using hemagglutination standards to measure EIA types of tests. So how should this adjustment be made?

DR. NAKAMURA: Are your people making purified antibody conjugates?

DR. TENOSO: No, we are not making purified conjugates.

DR. NAKAMURA: Dr. Wolfgang Becker of Behring Diagnostics has stated that his group is beginning to use purified antibody conjugates in their EIA systems. To reduce background and non-specific staining, one would prefer an enzyme-labeled conjugate to immunochemically purified $F(ab)_2$ or Fab antibody fragments.

DR. NAKANE: A subcommittee for enzyme-labeled antibody standards met in Stockholm in March 1978 to discuss the best way to define enzyme-labeled antibodies and develop a standard. The next meeting was held in Vienna in April 1978. There, the subcommittee that met consisted of representatives from five nations and there were two different opinions. One was that we should base the standard purely on a physiochemical definition and not use any given material. The other opinion was to designate a given material to be made available as a standard for comparison. The committee approved both options.

Approximately 30 companies that are members of charter of the World Health Organization have been contacted and asked to provide standard material. In other words, we are not interested in a procedure in which we have only 5mg of material that is used up in the characterization test. I have been informed that there are several companies which have adequate amounts of the enzyme-labeled antihuman IgG without specificity for light chains. The potency will be based on enzyme activity, and the antibody activity of the total solution will be defined as one. Also, just how much of the enzymatic activity is actually attached to an active antibody will be defined. Different laboratories will then evaluate the conjugates to determine whether the various methods may be interchangeable.

DR. NAKAMURA: How are you going to measure the antibody activity?

DR. NAKANE: This is going to be a peroxidase-labeled anti-human IgG. The peroxidase enzyme activity will be measured by standard methods converting H_2O_2 at 25°C. The antibody activity will be measured by the amount of enzyme which is attached to the solid state support. In other words, the antibody with attached enzyme is measured.

DR. TENOSO: Does that mean that in terms of time and availability, we are looking two years into the future?

DR. NAKANE: I hate to make a prediction, however we are supposed to have all preliminary members of the enzyme standards group complete the preliminary work by February 1979 and then meet to discuss the results.

DR. BEUTNER: Are we studying the competence of goats and rabbits and the competence of devout chemists, or are we studying human diseases?

If indeed we are more interested in the latter, the more appropriate reference standard might then be human sera. If you want to study immunoglobulin, serum protein levels, or specific antibody levels, the sera of patients are the appropriate reference calibrators. At the Vienna meeting, I felt that the compromise was not a well-advised one. What we need are well-standardized assay methods, and these are what we should be looking at. It doesn't seem appropriate to me that CAP or WHO or any other organization should go into competition with industry. Industry's need is for well-standardized methodology. I do feel that our dedication, since we are competent laboratory workers, should be to evaluating methods for studying conjugates. Once we have obtained some usable methods, it doesn't really matter whether we're using conjugates from the CAP or anyone else.

DR. SAUNDERS: I have a few general comments. Dr. Nakane mentioned that it would be nice if there were a test in which a stick could be used. The German workers have developed what they call stick ELISA. I'm not so sure how ELISA likes to be stuck, but the procedure involves one reagent being bound to a stick and being transferred to a series of tubes containing the patient's test sample and other necessary reagents.

The other comment concerns Dr. Paul Nakane's remark that it would be nice to use red blood cells in some kind of a vehicle to do these tests. Any of you who have worked with complement fixation tests know that there are many problems with the simple standardization of red blood cells. I can imagine the great problem one would have in standardizing blood cells as a vehicle to do EIA's. When I was doing the Jerne hemolytic plaque assays some time ago, one required the same sheep source and desired red cells of a certain age to maintain good quality control. Also, to the commercial companies, the bottom line is important with respect to the number of tests performed and the dollar value of those tests.

You know that in this country every year 100 million swine are slaughtered along with 50 million cattle and two billion chickens. Part of our research effort has been geared toward instituting EIA procedures to test cattle and swine for a series of four to five diseases as they go through the slaughter plant in order to protect the consumer and also as an epidemiological tool to trace pockets of important economic diseases. If the USDA ever gets to the point where they accept these tests, there will be a marketplace for the commercial manufacturers. Also, in veterinary practice in this country, cats and other pets should be tested for leukemia virus and canine heart worm. There would be a market for several million of these two tests per year. I hope the commercial companies would consider development of veterinary test products as well as for the tests for evaluation of human diseases.

DR. NAKANE: The use of erythrocytes may not be as difficult as discussed by Dr. Saunders. There is a way of subjecting red blood cells to permanent fixation yet leaving them susceptible to attack by complement. In addition, there is a way of using ghosts of red blood cells and incorporating compounds within the cell with formation of vesicles; these vesicles are also subject to the complement attack. These cellular particles are extremely stable and can be standardized against a reference preparation.

DR. SCHNEIDER: I would like to share a couple of ideas with you. First, a comment about erythrocyte ghosts. Our group has never been completely satisfied with the stability and performance characteristics of assays that use erythrocyte ghosts. In order to circumvent these problems, we prepared synthetic liposomes. When correctly made, these synthetic liposomes (vesicles) have good stability. If a vesicle is prepared in a medium which contains an enzyme, it is possible to encapsulate some of the enzyme inside the vesicle. A wide variety of enzymes have been encapsulated and the resulting vesicle used in an assay system. Analytical systems designed to use an enzyme encapsulated vesicle reagent generally are employed in assays where vesicle integrity is a function of phospholipase activity in the sample. When the vesicle is ruptured, the encapsulated enzyme is released. Amplification of sensitivity is attained through measurement of the freed enzyme. Through the use of a nonendogenous encapsulated enzyme, many of the problems of sample background can be eliminated.

Another comment concerns the previous discussion of screening tests by Dr. Saunders. There seems to be a genuine interest and need for qualitative assays, for a variety of drugs or natural compounds where screening for presence or absence of a compound is all that is required. The use of homogeneous enzyme immunoassay techniques may be ideally suited for such an application. Such assays would often not be performed by skilled technologists in a clinical laboratory. It becomes unrealistic to expect high precision and accuracy for a test of this type if pipetting and measuring steps are performed by relatively unskilled test users. In order to provide the necessary precision, reagents for immunoassays can be packaged in a single test form. The precision of reagent dispensing is assumed by the manufacturer. The user is only required to add the sample, mix the reagents, measure, and record the result. Single test formulations for such assays as glucose, lactic dehydrogenase, and cholesterol are already available for use in nonlaboratory environments, and there is no fundamental reason to preclude the use of homogeneous enzyme immunoassay reagents in an analogous way. If only qualitative or semiquantitative results are needed, so much the better.

DR. KEITGES: I just want to make two points. First, as president of the NCCLS, I would reassure Dr. Beutner that both the NCCLS and the College have firm Board-approved policies that they will never become involved in the business of manufacturing materials. Commercial manufacturers have asked these groups for specifications of standards. In the case of the digoxin assay, through a cooperative effort among the CDC, the NCCLS, and the AACC, the method almost dictated that a certain type of material would work best, so the standard will include not only a method, but a material. The industry then will produce the material, the CAP having no intention of manufacturing it.

The second point regards the same area. At the AACC meeting in San Francisco, Kodak introduced its answer to the Dupont ACA. Instead of cassettes, it uses film impregnated with the reagents, and the material is advanced in the machine to do the different tests in the same way that film is advanced in a camera. Now this is only for clinical chemistry, but from what I've heard referred to today, I could see a very definite application here.

DR. BEUTNER: I would like to thank NCCLS for the methodologies it has developed. I have participated on some of the subcommittees. It is unfortunate that some of the findings and recommendations of the NCCLS are being ignored at times, even by the WHO, which is reportedly turning out some of these reference standards which are competing with industry. I would like to see more of the findings and recommendations of NCCLS publicized. I think it is a gross error, absolutely ridiculous, for the WHO to compete with industry. I would really like to see it done outside of that organization. There has not been nearly enough cooperation between WHO and the NCCLS.

DR. KEITGES: There are two little lights on the gray cloud. One, we hope this meeting will be a pacesetter for recommendations. Also, the first meeting of the National Reference Systems in Clinical Chemistry under the aegis of the NCCLS will be held in Philadelphia next week, and that will be a joint effort by government, industry, and the professions to have totally voluntary consensus development of standards. We are looking forward to a tripartite agreement from the NBS, CDC, and the FDA, in which they are going to support in principle this voluntary development of standards.

Since we all admit that some of these standards will take years to develop, the FDA is interested in what the professions and industry think about the concept of parametric standards, which is really another name for more definitive specific labeling. The concept, very briefly, is that the professionals and government, working together with industry, would set criteria by which a new product would be judged. The manufacturer than would attach his label and the knowledgeable user could read it and determine if that product would meet his needs.

The FDA feels that it may get off the hook of all this Class 2 classification by using parametric standards. At some point in any of these four discipline areas we are going to discuss, perhaps a vote for or support of or a question mark for this concept of parametric standards should be considered.

Part III

DISCUSSION PERIOD

DR. CAVALLARO: To begin the discussion, it seems obvious, from the four papers we heard this morning, that despite the fact that immunofluorescence has been with us for 37 years, it still is an evolving complex area of investigation laden with much disagreement. One of the key notes that comes from these four papers is that perhaps the main crux of this whole conference has been standardization. Despite the fact that Dr. Nakamura told us of some new developments, we are still faced with the problem of standardization and proper controls. Similarly, the paper presented by Dr. Horan is exciting and presents a new application of immunofluorescence. Dr. Palmer has summarized very well the need for standardization.

I'd like to revert, however, to the definition given by Dr. Walls yesterday, which we sometimes lose sight of in standardizing a test. In standardizing a test, we are not only referring to standard reagents, conjugate, and proper controls, but we should also put these components together in a written format so that one can derive a methodology clearly spelled out with proper controls and reagents. Regarding Dr. Beutner's discussion about conjugates, and the fact that they should have a certain F:P ratio and antibody-to-protein ratio, as well as other defined criteria such as the optimal optical system—such standards will allow comparison of results from one laboratory to another and are badly needed.

Are there other comments?

DR. KEITGES: I've been told by people experienced in immunofluorescence that probably nowhere is the separation of things and people more important. One thing that we're talking about and hearing more and more about is standards of practice.

Maybe standards of practice are what are needed most in the average clinical laboratory doing immunofluorescence today. Of course, one should take into consideration some of the future advances, but for the everyday practice of immunofluorescence in the average clinical laboratory, we probably need some standards of practice and procedures. If a laboratory is going to do immunofluorescence, there are certain things that must be done in terms of how the test is set up and how the technologist gets it ready, using positive and negative controls to develop his or her answer. I've been appalled and fascinated by the originality that is exhibited by laboratories when we have inspected them in this area.

161

DR. CHANDOR: I'd like to emphasize what Dr. Keitges has said; not only does one have to worry about the antisera that one is dealing with, but also about the technologists and the tissue. The committee may want to deal with how to handle tissue and the kind of tissue to be used for immunofluorescent studies.

For instance, the clinicians pay a great deal of attention to the lupus band test. One wants to make sure that one has a great deal of confidence in doing the procedure because the clinician may make a diagnosis on that observation without serologic support. In renal biopsies a diagnosis of immune complex disease may be made if the fluorescence tests are positive regardless of what the light and electron microscopy may show. So it is important, as Dr. Keitges pointed out, to standardize not only the conjugate but also outline how the tissue specimens and sections in immunofluorescence are handled.

Another aspect of the tissue phase that Dr. Beutner brought up is that not only are we going to be dealing with immunofluorescence but also with the immunoperoxidase evaluation of tissue. In the future, this problem should be examined as to controls, antiserum, etc. The use of immunoperoxidase, especially with the PAP technique, is becoming a fairly widespread and popular procedure. We're starting to use it in a definitive way. Many of the cases that are sent to Dr. Lauren Ackerman for surgical pathology consultation at our institution are difficult, and to have tissue fluorescence or immunoperoxidase studies to demonstrate the cytoplasmic content of certain proteins or hormones can be very helpful. So in the future we may not only have to deal with tissue immunofluorescence problems, but also with problems associated with tissue immunoperoxidase assays.

DR. BEUTNER: I would submit the following for consideration as one means of coping with the problems at hand. Perhaps it would be best to focus on just one test system to break it down. For example, we could start with the immunofluorescent ANA test. The basic need of the clinical laboratory is to evaluate the relative reliability of a particular test. It seems unlikely that we will be able to dictate to manufacturers the type of kits they turn out, nor will it be possible for us to dictate to laboratories which manufacturer's kit to buy. Perhaps our reference laboratory (International Service for Immunology Laboratories) could be of service and make available a series of three SLE sera along with a series of three normal control sera.

Allow me to digress for a moment to consider the nature of the disease process and the relationship of the immune response to the disease process under study. There is a wide variability in autoimmune responses in different cases of SLE. The ANA level is usually elevated. However, there are, despite all protestations to the contrary, SLE cases that are ANA negative. They need not be in crisis; these are simply individuals whose particular immunologic abnormalities do not include ANA. Secondly, ANA do occur in normal sera. In fact, low ANA titers may play the role of normal physiologic responses. In other words, we are dealing here with a spectrum ranging from normal responses to those seen in SLE. Obviously, we must evaluate the range of normal values and of the significance of ANA in SLE.

No one ANA test system is going to be 100% perfect as a diagnostic aid in SLE. As previously indicated, we have sera in volume, and data on at least three known SLE cases with a range of high, medium and low ANA titers, and different patterns. We should send these to all laboratories that care to evaluate them. The data could be subject to a breakdown of the type that Dr. Palmer has described for the toxoplasma assay, that is, in terms of particular manufacturer, their substrates and conjugates, and the particular optimal system used to read them.

In tissue immunofluorescence there is a real weakness in the titration of immunofluorescence tests, notably the optical sensitivity of fluorescence microscopes. Different types of microscopes and filters yield divergent readings. We cannot dictate to the clinical laboratory which microscope to use, nor which particular set of filters and objectives to use, nor how workers will align their microscopes. What laboratories need for immunofluorescence work is simple set standard reference slides with microdroplets of fluorescein at a range of known concentrations. Such standard reference slides could be prepared at a modest price and could be made readily available to laboratories for evaluation of the relative sensitivity of their optical system.

DR. RITCHIE: I think we might be running the risk of designing another camel, and you all know how the camel came into being. The reason I think we run this risk, and would be vulnerable to some fairly incisive complaints, is that we have, within the CAP and other organizations in the country, a fair amount of expertise but we make use of it out of the good offices and generosity of individual laboratories and their directors. There is no active program whereby Dr. Beutner's comments could be brought in under the fold. We have a management system and an administrative system, but we have no laboratory system as a part of CAP's efforts.

I think that we might consider designing a structure whereby expert laboratories become part of the CAP's effort. We have all the paperwork, but we don't have the machinery. In a way, we have all the marketing and sales effort, but we don't have the production. The procedures Dr. Beutner just described, of testing out the materials and the methods by which the materials are evaluated, and the instruments on which they are being tested, should be part of that effort. So that when we sit down here as a group of individuals trying to standardize laboratory medicine, we could hear from someone who is part of our organization, who has contacted other experts in their specific area, and who can give us a relatively unbiased opinion. I think it's worth considering.

For example, there are laboratories in this country that do anti-nuclear antibody studies by the thousands. Some of the people who direct those laboratories also have an interest in research and are part of the CAP. Wouldn't it be helpful to a laboratory under our collective guidance, in your own laboratory for example, to evaluate some of the things that Dr. Beutner has just outlined and to set up a well-designed program of internal quality control?

DR. KEITGES: The College is sponsoring a doctoral position in clinical chemistry at the National Bureau of Standards for this very purpose. These problems would be directed to that individual, who has the tremendous resources of the NBS at his disposal. I think you've hit upon a very interesting concept. The same problems are present in other areas, such as microbiology and hematology, and the funding of positions in various disciplines would be very expensive. But I find the concept extremely interesting.

DR. DEODHAR: The CAP also supports a standards laboratory which at present is located at Cleveland Clinic, but as I understand it, the support is for certain equipment and one technologist. Perhaps, with better supervisory control, the activities of this laboratory could be expanded to include the type of things about which we are talking.

DR. KEITGES: I would think, for example, that such a distinguished group as this should come out with some recommendations of that kind for implementation. There is such a wealth of data, and I'm sure the CDC has the same situation with their proficiency testing data. Regarding Dr. Beutner's concept of sending out these known or unknown samples, in a way this is being done every other month in the CAP Survey Programs. We should start thinking about determining just how much information is in that data. I know that Dr. Bowman, chairman of the CAP Diagnostic Immunology Resource Committee, has been trying to assign certain areas of analysis and review of data to different individuals on his committee.

DR. CAVALLARO: I think the point is very well taken. We already have the answers for most of the questions that have arisen regarding standardization. As Dr. Keitges mentioned, we have the data, and perhaps if a body such as this, CDC, or others, promulgated and recorded these recommendations, the adaptation would be facilitated. Because, as we were discussing, it is not uncommon to receive questions about which is the best standard substrate to use. For instance, in IF-ANA, most people would recommend mouse liver, but there is another side; most people would agree, but it's not written down. F:P ratios are similar.

DR. KEITGES: I would like to ask a question about that. It was mentioned that there should be a standard procedure for determining an F:P ratio. All laboratories doing immunofluorescence should know this standard procedure.

DR. BEUTNER: The NCCLS has set forth recommendations on procedures for determining fluorescence and protein, and the calculations are grocery store arithmetic. Again, I would like to raise the banner of the NCCLS and promote its recommendations vigorously. We have followed these recommendations and found them to be quite satisfactory with good reproducibility. There are very few problems if the procedures are done conscientiously with appropriate reference standards.

DR. KEITGES: I'm aware of that. However, the laboratories must be encouraged to adopt a good standard practice and procedure as outlined by NCCLS. You're right, it exists, but many laboratories are not following the NCCLS recommendations.

DR. BEUTNER: Perhaps the ISIL could contribute here. We have detailed write-ups of the entire methodologies. Indeed, we want to submit these for consideration by the CAP.

DR. NAKAMURA: The proposal is for a standardized IF-ANA test, similar to the syphilis serology test in which there is a standard procedure, with controls of high and low positive sera and negative sera with the standard reagents. The big problem in the autoantibody test is positive controls. In the IF-ANA test, one wants to have a high and low titered positive control sera. The low titer sera will be useful to define the test in the detection of low affinity antibody. Chessboard titrations on every fluorescent reagent pool should be done with both low and high titered positive sera. These control sera will help in maintaining consistency and reproducibility. Also, the substrate tissue sections should be of uniform size, and a definite amount of serum dilutions and conjugate should be placed on the sections in the test procedure.

DR. SCHNEIDER: Not being an immunologist by training, I am really an observer to a group such as this. Saying this allows me to make some statements giving a layman's conception of your current concerns. I wrote down some thoughts and tried to define to myself what you're talking about.

It appears that fluorescence assays are really divided into

two distinct types. One is a serum measurement. The other type of assay is a tissue measurement. My observation has been that, in tissue fluorescence measurements, there are large variations introduced by the equipment (e.g. the microscope, the mounting, the size of the section), the preparation of the tissue, and the preparation of the immunochemical reagents. All are independent variables, and these are hard to control. The tests and results are extremely technique-oriented. Reagents can often be homemade. Some are available in kits, but often they are not. Results often depend on someone's objectivity in reading a microscope or in interpreting something observed. Dr. Beutner said that tissue immunologists should have some kind of standard; that is, for example, fluorescein embedded in a plastic matrix. It seems to me that with tissue fluorescence measurements, the need for standardized procedures is also very important. With a standardized procedure comes the need for controls and proficiency samples.

Now contrast the state of tissue measurements with that of serum or fluid measurements utilizing a fluorescence technique. Very often, instruments are used to measure the sample, to monitor a reaction, and to record the result. The subjectivity encountered with tissue measurements is avoided through instrumentation. One is not subjecting somebody's eyes to being calibrated. Reagents are generally commercially provided, so that much of the variation in reagent preparation is greatly diminished. Commercial reagents are not always of the best quality, but much of the reagent variation is limited because there are fewer reagent companies than there are laboratories making their own reagents. Tests are often automated. This takes much of the individual's technical ability and personal variation out of the procedure. It seems to me that in the case of serum and liquid measurements, the need for a standardized procedure isn't so great. There is an enormous need for standardized controls; that is, negative, low, medium, and high result-oriented material. However, the procedure itself doesn't matter so much.

To summarize very quickly, there are two types of measurements that you're concerned with as pathologists. One is tissue fluorescence measurements, and the other is serum or liquid measurements. I think we ought to try to divide our thinking along these lines rather than lumping everything together and try to come out with a series of generalized recommendations. I think that by dividing, you have a chance to conquer; whereas, if we condense everything together, only confusion will result.

DR. RITCHIE: It's always nice to hear an organized mind address something that is relatively new. We probably make greater steps that way than in any other. I think your last comment about dividing and conquering is to the point. I refer to my statement just a moment ago that dividing the individuals who are available to us and coopting them as experts with their laboratories behind them is the way to address such problems. I think certain expert laboratories should address the problems.

Most of the issues we've talked about today, if addressed properly, present arduous tasks, boring and expensive, that nobody really wants to do. When we're faced with a situation of asking the question, for example, "What is the range of IgG in a population?" nobody wants to address it. It just happens that we had a computer to do it. I think almost everything we've talked about today is boring work to most people. If you can't narrow it down and break it into pieces so that a specific laboratory knowledgeable in the area can address it efficiently, we're never going to get it done. I agree with Dr. Schneider that the only way to handle it is to divide and conquer.

DR. NAKANE: There is considerable confusion here. Certain people have emphasized procedures, and I'm not quite sure if that's the thing to be emphasized. Essentially, what is really important is performance and not necessarily standardized procedures. When one has a given serum, one wants to know if it is a positive or not. That's what you're asking. What kind of a microscope is used or what kind of an eyeball is used isn't important. If it's a positive, it's a positive; if it's a negative, it's a negative. So therefore, what it really comes down to is that the procedure is of secondary importance. What we should always think about ultimately are the performance specifications.

A question may arise when one laboratory will report a positive and another laboratory will report a negative result on the same specimen. That's where the problem starts. Certain people have argued that we need reference standards, one of which will be positive, another, negative. It's probably one of the possible approaches, but I'm just asking questions because the standardization of a procedure is not important.

DR. NAKAMURA: That's what we want—a control sera with high and low values which are well characterized.

DR. NAKANE: And if you use that sera, no matter what procedure you use, if it becomes a positive that's fine, and if it gives a control of negative that's fine.

DR. KEITGES: One thing that has really impressed me, especially since I got into this position of being in charge of a national system for developing laboratory standards, is the tremendous limit to our resources. The government, industry, and the professions realize that there is a limit to the amount of people, time, and money we have to do these things. I feel that merely following the quest of accuracy and precision without considering clinical relevance and medical usefulness could be a serious error because of the limit to our resources.

Therefore, I think we need combined efforts, not just a laboratory but a combined group, and I would just like to offer one example which I think may not be "*the* model," but *a* model. I am referring to the recent contract the FDA gave to the NCCLS for the anaerobic antimicrobial susceptibility testing project. Here are ten laboratories, each contributing its expertise: an institution contributing the organism, a company contributing the culture media, the plates, etc., the government contributing the funds to support the ten laboratories. They are meeting in Denver today, and the testing has started.

The committee met and designed a reference protocol for anaerobic antimicrobial susceptibility testing. They will now test that protocol, using organisms and a standardized culture media, and see what they come up with. It may be unsuccessful, but it may result in a reference method for this testing such as Kirby-Bauer. The point I'm trying to make is, and I think Dr. Sommers would agree, that there's a real clinical need for some sort of standardization there.

DR. WALLS: I'm disturbed by this "Let's just do something, and if we get a positive it's positive, and if we get a negative it's negative." I'm in the same position as Dr. Schneider—I'm not associated with a hospital so I can speak from ignorance. I get telephone calls almost daily from clinicians wanting to know what the reported titer of a test means. If all I can say is, "Well it was compared to a standard and it was positive," I can't help him at all. I've got to be able to tell him that yes, a titer of 1:1024 has some meaning, and the report that you obtain from me has the same meaning as the one you receive from your state health department.

The IUSIS got involved in the standardization of EIA about two years ago when the test was virtually unused. There were only a dozen laboratories even playing with it. But the whole principle of getting involved was that immunofluorescence was in a mess because they waited fifteen years to get into the field and everybody was doing it their way; they were making their conjugates their way, they were making their standards this way and that way. And now they've got all this mess together.

If we start off by saying, "Go ahead and do it any way you want, gang; we'll give you some controls and then ten years from now we're going to make you all come back together," then we have a real problem. If we start looking now at specific standards, we have a better chance of not ending up ten years from now in a hodgepodge of techniques that have to all be "standardized" against what one laboratory says: "This is my technique and it's the best," or another that says: "This is my technique, that's the best." So I think we can't start off "sloppy." We have to start out with some specifics. Perhaps standard serum, because you have to start somewhere.

DR. SOMMERS: Dr. Walls has a very good point. We all agree that we should start preparing standard immunologic reagents of some kind, but I question if it is necessary to have such standards in hand before we can start an interlaboratory survey on different types of procedures. The surveys can contribute a great deal to establishing and validating an optimal test method or procedure. We have had experience in this area with antimicrobial susceptibility testing in the microbiology surveys.

To perform the Bauer-Kirby antimicrobial susceptibility test in a consistent and reproducible manner, there are a number of clearly defined steps that should be taken to control a series of variables that may have a significant effect on the interpretation of the test. Not all clinical microbiology laboratories follow these steps. By means of a questionnaire, we were able to identify a subset of participants who followed these guidelines in contrast to those who did not. Performance of laboratories following the guidelines was significantly more consistent in the zone of growth inhibition and the interpretation of results than participants who did not make the extra effort.

I am sure that your own group can set up and collect information by an interlaboratory comparison survey that can be of great help in establishing standard reagents and procedures. Experience gained in comparison surveys during the time reagents are being standardized will make the validation of such reagents and procedures much more simple when they are available. There will also be considerable information available from previous comparison surveys that can be of significant help.

DR. NAKAMURA: The one question that I always ask is: "What is the criteria for specificity of the reagents to be used in the fluorescence immunoassays?" In 1969, when the organization met to set criteria for specificity of immunofluorescent reagents, the criteria was based on immunoelectrophoresis with a uniform homogeneous precipitin line. All of you that have been doing fluorescence obviously know that the light chains are going to cross react and not precipitate and that the precipitin reaction is a poor criteria for specificity. There are reagents which are specific for IgG and specific for free light chains by the criteria of immunoelectrophoresis. But you can't transfer the specificity of a precipitin reaction to a primary binding fluorescence reaction. We should use antigen-linked beads or some primary binding reaction to test the specificity of the fluorescent-labeled reagents.

In regard to the clinical relevance of IF-ANA, there are certain diseases that are negative by standard indirect tissue immunofluorescence tests, i.e. 50% of the cases of scleroderma and Sjögren's syndrome. Some of the antibody to some nuclear antigens are EB viral-related antigens. I think the idea of establishing controls for the participants to see how they're doing with their procedure is good. However, I would like to recommend that we come up with some recommendations for specificity and performance of immunochemical reagents in specific procedures.

DR. CAWLEY: I'd like to take a small exception to the thesis that we need to eliminate a mess in immunofluorescence. We have shown repeatedly that the majority of laboratories have come up with comparable results; by comparable results we mean, within reasonably narrow ranges. Titers are important; positive and negative are associated with the clinical interpretation.

I would also like to submit that we also separate the reproducibility of the laboratory test as one thing to achieve within a majority of laboratories. Secondly, having achieved some measure of reproducibility in terms of titers in the laboratory test, comes the question: What is the significance clinically? We must report a positive or a negative control with known values and diseases. With IF-ANA for example, it is possible to achieve a reproducible system under reasonably refined conditions. It is also possible for us to start to build the second step confirming ANA titers, and correlation with clinical conditions and diseases.

DR. CHANDOR: I'd like to make a comment about the positive and negative controls. I think we have to be prepared to give guidelines as to their preparation. The rheumatoid factor assay, as pointed out by Dr. Horan, could show the difference between how the control is prepared and how the lab prepares the patient serum. If a positive control has been heated, and you don't tell the laboratory to heat patient's sera, they're likely to get entirely different results, and the control will be worthless as far as dealing with their patient sample. So I think that not only do we need the controls, but also some basic guidelines on how to handle a specific test so that the control and the patient's material are handled in the same manner.

DR. SCHNEIDER: I think we have to keep in mind what kind of question we are asking before trying to grab for an answer. For instance, the question, "Does a person have syphilis or is the woman pregnant?" can be answered with a qualitative response. It's classic that you can't be a little positive in either of those conditions. If you need to know the extent of pregnancy, all that is required is a visual observation. Observation in this case really isn't too bad. On the other hand, to ask the question, "Does somebody have immunoglobulin G?" and to answer "yes" or "no" seems ridiculous. Here, one needs quantitation in order to provide a meaningful result. I was thinking about the question of whether or not a qualitative response is useful. Yes, sometimes it's very useful. Sometimes it isn't. If you can better define which question belongs in which category, you can probably provide an answer with less ambiguity.

DR. CAVALLARO: I'd like to make a statement, though, that there are times, especially in infectious diseases, where we do want a titer, we do want to quantitate! It may make the difference between treatment or no treatment, and in that aspect I think we do want quantitation as Dr. Walls mentioned. So a simple yes or no answer may be of no use.

Part IV

DISCUSSION PERIOD

DR. HURTUBISE: To begin, and to discuss briefly what the various speakers have described to you, I would like to reiterate a very simple concept. We in the clinical laboratory are presented with a specimen which may represent a tissue, cells in peripheral blood, or serum. It has been submitted to us so that we can make a determination as to whether a patient does or does not have a disease. This is an oversimplification, but we must talk about a qualitative, as well as a quantitative, type of testing.

In the area of immunology, most of the tests with which we deal are not "stat" tests, but represent part of a cluster of tests to define a specific disease state. In fact, Dr. Rose indicated that there are some groupings of diseases where cellular immunology tests do have important clinical value, at least in terms of defining a disease state. Again, an oversimplified list is probably a series of six or seven categories for which we test. I might comment that in the in vitro testing we do, at least in the cellular immunology area of immunodeficiency states, significant results are seen in the frank immunodeficiency states. The subtle immunodeficiency states are difficult to find, and we do not have adequate tools with which to correctly evaluate these conditions. We have done very little in the area of infectious diseases, one of the areas that should be more extensively explored. Consider, for example, the patient as a compromised host with infections. It is becoming increasingly evident, as chemotherapeutic agents are used, that many of our patients are dying—not because of their cancer—but because of infection.

With respect to autoimmune diseases, I have asked Dr. Daniels to make some comments because he has data of clinical relevance related to the use of cellular immunology tests in autoimmune diseases.

Lymphoproliferative malignancy is an extensive area that has been studied. Data generated in this area defines whether a malignancy is or is not present. One can use peripheral blood in leukemic states as well as bone marrow or other tissues. Tumor immunology has probably advanced the whole area of cellular immunology and its applications. Many researchers are now reevaluating and reexamining the various cellular tests in tumor immunology.

173

The area of allergy and drug allergies, as indicated by Dr. Barna, is one that is providing information.

One of the very specific areas that I like to lump together is that which I call protocol medicine. Dr. Rose indicated that this may be an area of fruitful examination for us. One would examine the beginning stages of the disease to establish a good baseline and then monitor the patient for relative changes which may occur. This may be more relevant than looking at clusters of diseases.

A couple of problems in terms of standardization of methodology between laboratories have been brought to my attention. Probably the greatest existing stumbling block for cellular assay is the lack of decent methods for transporting cellular material between laboratories. If we are going to consider interlaboratory data, I believe this is one of the areas into which we must look.

We should point out that there are several resources available on methodology. One is an excellent manual on clinical immunology printed by the American Society of Microbiology and edited by Dr. Rose and Dr. Friedman. The CDC has recently produced a good manual for doing B- and T-cell assays. I am aware that the southwest and southeast oncology groups have attempted to standardize some of these procedures within their own groups so that their data will become more meaningful.

Finally, I think that large institutions with extensive experience are very valuable resources in this area. This point was brought up by Dr. Rose at the conclusion of his talk.

Another problem with standardization of the tests centers on the question, "What are generally acceptable criteria for defining a lymphocyte or a macrophage?" This represents a serious problem. I'd like to ask Dr. Daniels to speak now about his experience with cellular tests in autoimmune diseases.

DR. DANIELS: I'd like to preface my remarks by saying that when one wanders into the world of cell-mediated immunity, one encounters a variety of tests which look terribly intriguing, and is tempted to measure everything simply because one *can* measure it. Here I think a theme that has been apparent throughout the conference can be highlighted. We are faced with a variety of technical procedures which are virtually unstandardized. No one would question that. Then we're faced with the ultimate question that was posed the first day: So what? One is forced to consider the question of clinical relevance, more in the area of cell-mediated immune tests than in some of the other areas we have discussed. We must know clearly and pointedly why we're going to perform a test if indeed a patient is going to be charged for that service. It's great intellectual fun to think through the immune system and to go into the laboratory and measure things because they can be measured. But if we're going to approach the bedside and make clinical decisions in cell-mediated immunity, we must know what question we are asking. Here, even the idea of qualitative versus quantitative tests becomes blurred because, as Dr. Rose pointed out, one can have significant intralaboratory correlation, but due to lack of standardization (and I think it will be quite some time before we have that standardization), one does not have acceptable interlaboratory correlation. If you can agree with yourself all of the time, you can get highly quantitative results, but the quantitation at the bottom line comes out being a plus or a minus, so that even the concepts of qualitative versus quantitative testing become blurred in certain areas.

We have numerous ways of approaching the immune system, very much as Dr. Rose pointed out, dissecting first the morphology and then the function. It would be quite inappropriate to perform a total immunological dissection in a given case other than for research, except perhaps in exceedingly rare cases. On a service basis one *must* ask a specific question. What do you want to know? It's good to have an assay that you at least have faith in and can agree with yourself on, though you may not agree with another laboratory because of the lack of standards. This is a circuitous way of getting around to making some remarks based on Dr. Hurtubise's comments that autoimmunity is one of the clinically relevant areas for the application of cell-mediated immunoassays.

The rosette assays that we've already heard about for T- and B-cell enumeration have been taken a step further, as many people here know, to subpopulations of T-helper and T-suppressor lymphocytes. Functional cell types have very specific markers on the surface. The T-helper cells have a receptor for immunoglobulin M, and therefore, these are called Tμ cells. Other cells, Tγ as they're called, have a receptor for IgG, and these are the T-suppressor lymphocytes. So one can dissect out T-helper or T-suppressor cells simply by doing a double rosette technique in which you first obtain enriched T-lymphocytes and then see if they will react as rosettes with erythrocytes coated with either IgG or IgM.

In using this approach, designating the shorthand system that Tγ are the suppressor cells and Tμ are the helper cells, we find that according to current dogma one can demonstrate in the laboratory that Tγ cells in systemic lupus erythematosus patients are indeed decreased, while the Tμ cells, or the helper cells, are quite normal. That is, there is a decrease in T-suppressor cell number, as well as function, in these SLE patients.

Why does this have clinical relevance? It's an admixture, in a way, of Dr. Hurtubise's classification of protocol medicine in that there are thymosin extracts that one can give under FDA-approved protocol to restore Tγ function. We are studying this now and we believe lymphocyte subset enumeration correlates with restoration of Tγ function in patients with SLE. Of course, in these SLE patients it may take five years of follow-up to develop an impression of whether administration of thymosin, which is effective in restoring T-suppressor function, is contributory to clinical improvement. But Tγ and Tμ lymphocyte measurement has clinical relevance in that we can select patients who are candidates for this immunological replacement therapy. We can follow the success or failure of thymosin therapy, and we think it has prognostic value. This is on the verge of being both the present and the future.

DR. CHANDOR: The point has been made that there are numerous tests, and the establishment of good quality control on these cellular tests between laboratories is unlikely in the near future. Something that can be done, as Dr. Rose pointed out, is to give some guidance to laboratories that are performing these tests and try to determine whether all mitogens, or just one or two, are needed, and which immunoglobulin on the cell surface defines a B-cell. Should Fab antisera be used instead of whole molecule antisera? These questions should be resolved.

Dr. Rose pointed out that many of the patients have recurrent and persistent infections. Therefore, besides doing a white count differential, should one test for the function of the polymorphonuclear leukocytes (NBT test, phagocytosis, killing)? Such procedures play a role in the clinical immunology laboratory, such as in the diagnosis of chronic granulomatous diseases. Also, many patients are seen because they have rheumatology problems, especially back pain. One of the tests that clinicians frequently request is HLA typing. All this appears to be a part of clinical immunology.

DR. RITZMANN: I think the contribution by Dr. Daniels regarding the better diagnostic and etiopathogenic understanding of SLE is a very appropriate topic. Dr. Yoshida mentioned the quantitation of lymphokines using the RIA technique. We can probably learn a lesson from the methodology applied to drug screening, where one method, e.g. liquid chromatography, is utilized for the measurement or detection of numerous different drugs. Perhaps the principle of this approach, with its inherent high sensitivity, should be considered as a practical approach for the assay of lymphokines.

DR. KEITGES: I was very impressed by Dr. Rose's remarks on normality. I would like to give you a brief model that I think may be a valuable tool in this field to help us bring closer together this continual imbalance between accuracy and precision on one hand and clinical relevance on the other. It's the so-called retrospective clinical study from which you evaluate your numbers in terms of their meaning.

This study was done by Dr. Cole at the University of Alabama. He simply labeled a thousand females admitted to the University of Alabama over a finite period of time, accepting the fact that the normal BUN was 10-20. You would expect a Gaussian distribution of about that so-called normal range. His philosophy, by the way, is that we should stop worrying about normals. What is important is what he calls clinically useful ranges. Using a retrospective study, a thousand charts were reviewed by residents and himself. It took hundreds of hours. They found a small hump in the 18-28mg/100ml range. And in that group of females, more than 30% had significant renal disease and no clinical symptoms. So in that institution and that population anyone with a BUN from 18-28 should undergo further study for occult renal disease, even to the point of including basic procedures because there was such a high incidence of undetected renal disease that it is clinically demanded.

All of us don't have the time to sit down and examine a thousand charts, but apparently a modification of the Bottachari technique for evaluating how many humps there are in a big hump is called a gram charlea technique. The CAP has now embarked upon a normal values project in which they are asking laboratories to send in 1,000 or 2,000 sodiums and then submitting those numbers to this gram charlea technique, a computerized formula. The preliminary studies are quite exciting; theoretically the technique detects these clinically significant humps within a so-called normal distribution. I think nothing cries more for this sort of approach than many of these findings we are generating in the field of immunology because we just don't know what their clinical relevance is. It seems as though we need that information first rather than afterward, and then maybe we would see areas in which we need to follow up.

DR. HURTUBISE: I think we will conclude with those remarks. You can all understand the confusion when you read Plato in the caves and they are discussing the shadows on the wall, trying to make sweeping conclusions from them. We are doing the same here this afternoon. Thank you.

DISCUSSION: SUMMATION and CONCLUSIONS

DR. KEITGES: I'd like to convene the final, and perhaps most important, session of this seminar on diagnostic immunology. We have had two days of excellent discussion.

This seminar was conceived by some of us who felt a very definitive and critical need in the discipline of diagnostic immunology. It was the consensus of opinion that a group of national experts be brought together to discuss this need. The philosophy was to address it in four aspects: immunoprecipitin techniques, immunofluorescence, enzyme label immunoassay, and cellular immunity.

We need to examine our present status and set up some specific goals. We can provide the leadership needed in establishing quality control in standards for the clinical laboratory.

This morning the four chairmen convened and by consensus have drafted what they consider to be a capsule paragraph which summarizes the important points.

It can be stated that in any immunologic procedure, the immunochemical reagents should be defined in terms of performance and specificity in a definitive immunological reaction. Performance may be defined in either qualitative and/or quantitative terms, but it must have clinical relevance.

The concepts of performance and specificity must be based on a common denominator of clinical relevance. Deliberation among the four chairmen revealed some confusion. As we became very excited about the dialogue, we noted a slight variation in terms being used, such as "control, assay, reference, standard, and procedure." A recommendation was then made that a glossary be developed. This is particularly fascinating to me, in that the clinical chemists have stated that there is a very real need for a glossary which is accepted and understood by clinicians and clinical chemists. It is proposed that an ad hoc committee (task force) be established to develop such a glossary for those clinicians and clinical chemists using immunological procedures.

We are also in agreement that there is a real need for leadership. Leadership, in this context, is best defined as a combined task force approach which would consider our limited resources, expertise, funds, time, and people. This was best summarized by Dr. Ritchie who stated that we must have a means of generating resources. Initially, funds should be obtained from an appropriate source; expertise should then be exploited in a plurality fashion. The existing vehicles

179

for this are obvious and we'd be mad to "re-invent the wheel." The Diagnostic Immunology Resource Committee of the CAP could establish protocols for this kind of task force or combined study approach. The NCCLS is an organization useful in an area where consensus is needed. The CDC has already been involved with a tremendous interest and capability. The Diagnostic Immunology Resource Committee of the CAP, the NCCLS, and the CDC could work cooperatively in seeking solutions to the problems or questions which have been raised.

The immunochemical reagent in any immunological procedure should be defined in terms of the performance and the specificity required in a definitive immunological reaction. The specificity required in indirect immunofluorescent tests is going to be very different from the specificity required in some of the esoteric cell-mediated immunity procedures. One of the problems we encounter is the practice of taking a reagent and saying, "Gee, if it works over here, we ought to be able to use it over here." That is madness! Specificity and performance are not only defined in terms of immunological reaction and whether it be immunoprecipitin or fluorescent. They are also defined in terms which can be either qualitative and/or quantitative, but there must be a common denominator or a relationship to clinical relevance. This was well summarized by Dr. Rose when he stated that certain immunoassays should not be standardized and enshrined, but should be left to eventually die a natural death. This is a very general philosophical approach, but I think it probably sets the tone of the proceedings.

Let us look now at control materials. Because of the marked difference in materials one must use in immunoprecipitin techniques versus cell-mediated immunity or enzyme label assays, we thought that at this point it would be appropriate to hear the chairmen's reports, since they will vary tremendously from area to area.

IMMUNOPRECIPITIN TECHNIQUES

The theme of the input here was centered around procedures and/or methods and materials. There is a definite concern about the need for definition, standardization, and prioritization of procedures and materials. In this area, performance and specificity are the hallmarks of efforts which should be undertaken to define what is needed in terms of both performance and clinical need; one can then proceed with regard to bringing more standardization, quality control, and specificity, not only to the materials used, but to their application and interpretation.

One recommendation that was introduced is the development of a secondary control serum that would be immediately referable and transferable to the primary standard which is currently being developed and approved by the World Health Organization through the International Union of Immunological Societies (IUIS), the so-called candidate preparation number three from Dr. Reimer at the CDC. This secondary standard will initially be used to establish commonality of the interlaboratory comparisons in proficiency testing.

If it is as fruitful and productive as we expect it to be, its use beyond that would certainly be appropriate. This secondary standard, which is being investigated and developed by the CAP, would be produced by industrial contract.

The initial goal is the immunoglobulins C3 and C4, AG and M, IgA, IgM, and IgG. Dr. Reimer believes that other proteins certainly should be evaluated from this same pool.

DR. RITCHIE: We have been hindered in assigning a mass unit to any control with plasma proteins because the state of the art is constantly evolving. What we did with the World Health Organization ten years ago is now viewed with a jaundiced eye. Technology has improved, and we can do a better job this time. There will be those who continue to procrastinate. I feel that it is time now to make some sort of philosophic statement concerning the assignment of a mass unit based upon the state of the art today. Otherwise, we will jump ahead year by year and end with nothing.

QUESTION FROM THE FLOOR: Will there be consideration in establishing this reference of terms for subclass specificity or homogeneity? This becomes important in measuring abnormal protein.

DR. NAKAMURA: In general, it can be assayed for subclass concentration of immunoglobulins. We are going to try to get a normal pool. What you are saying is, "What subclasses are in the normal pool, in case we want to evaluate it as a standard for subclass quantitation of immunoglobulins?" Dr. Ritchie stated that we should establish mass units in relation to the current state of the art, which means that the WHO units must be reevaluated because of the newer nephelometry techniques. When we consulted with Dr. Reimer, he felt that the only way the problem of the mass units could be settled was to find a reputable person who could actually produce 20mg of this chemically purified material to be used as a primary standard. Establishing these mass units at the current state of the art still poses a problem. If a pooled serum were to be purchased and assayed by means of a known, bona fide standard, we would then have a tertiary standard. Perhaps mass units could be established with an acceptable standard, validated by a survey, and thus become a consensus standard.

DR. RITCHIE: Perhaps it should be the task of the group to establish methods by which a purified material could be used for recovery studies. How pure and stable a material can be prepared today for this study? If we wait longer, I am not sure that we are going to get better results. Five years ago, six laboratories were asked to assay for the immunoglobulins in a candidate, and at that time, their results were so close that there was essentially no difference among them.

Dr. Nakamura, I propose that we develop a pool or different pools of control sera and make an effort to assign gravimetric units with the current state of the art under the direction of this leadership task force committee.

DR. KILLINGSWORTH: We must take some initial steps, and we are all interested in immunoglobulins C3 and C4, but I want to put in my bid for going a bit further. Then, defining how much further we go could be discussed at another time.

DR. NAKAMURA: We may be able to obtain a pool from Atlantic Antibodies and can assign values for 12 proteins. Do you think that this is a logical way to go?

DR. KILLINGSWORTH: It is a good idea. We should take the proteins that make up 95% of the mass of the serum proteins and start with those. If we want to get more esoteric, we can do that later.

DR. KEITGES: I'd like to reassure you a bit at this point. When Dr. Nakamura and I met with Dr. Reimer at CDC, we were advised to explore obtained primary standard purified material for a few of the common proteins. However, the standard pool can be expanded to include many proteins. The question was specifically, "What are we going to start with, and I think you are making sure that the door is kept open in the back."

I'd also like to mention that the task force concept is really taking over and catching on. I think this is excellent, and we are going to assume that the members of this conference will be willing volunteers for many of these conferences, in some cases as the chairmen. This will insure that our present endeavor stays on course.

DR. SAVORY: In my recommendation, I propose that we consider in detail the efforts of the International Federation of Clinical Chemists. The Expert Board on Proteins is working on standardization of albumin, IgG, IgA, IgM, and possibly also transferrin, orosomucoid, alpha-1-antitrypsin, and C3. Dr. Chester Alper is a member on the Expert Board on Proteins, and I am an associate member. I am sure we could profit by integrating our efforts with the IFCC.

DR. KEITGES: This would be appropriate. Dr. Alper called me just before this conference, and introduced the whole concept. Very briefly, the CAP is "beefing up" its international relationships, and the NCCLS now has formal international diplomatic liaison. Dr. Alper stated that as far as actually writing the standards, they would not even begin in their group in the IFCC, but would like this to be a voluntary consensus mechanism. I assure you that what they are doing will be taken into serious consideration as we develop this.

DR. BEUTNER: One of the important plasma proteins is fibrin; you have spoken here of serum. Is there any possibility of converting this into plasma so that fibrin can be included?

DR. KEITGES: This is exactly Dr. Nakamura's goal. He feels that if we had a plasma base material, we'd have much more flexibility than we would with a serum base material. Preparation number three is serum, but as Dr. Reimer said, this was merely easier to study. Dr. Reimer sees no reason why it could not be expanded to plasma—they just did not collect it as plasma. It was a fairly arbitrary decision on their part.

DR. NAKAMURA: When we first started, we wanted plasma because we wanted preservation of complement activity. The IUIS committee on complement standards used serum and wanted a functional standard as well as an immunochemical standard. Many of us would be happy with a good immunochemical standard. The committee has produced some good serum standards with preservation of complement activity. However, certain lots of serum were not good, and plasma is easier to collect and maintain complement activity than serum.

DR. HURTUBISE: When you develop a new standard, please develop it in terms of clinically high and clinically low values, because in each of the procedures dealt with in our massive studies, the instrumentation varied in performance when we were dealing with high values as opposed to low values. High and low values are very important for those of us in the laboratory.

DR. NAKAMURA: Essentially, three standards are preferable, because these standards should be established in relation to clinical relevance. Is it possible to develop such a range of good standards?

DR. RITCHIE: Our experience is that 1× and 3× concentrates of serum can be prepared with relative ease, but plasma standards are something else. The focus today is on serum with plasma in the background. The major constituent of the interest in plasma is fibrinogen, and since it is so easily and precisely assayed by non-immunochemical methods today, there really is no reason to devote much attention to a plasma standard.

DR. NAKAMURA: I would like to recommend that if this CAP group is going to make a standard or control sera available, that we provide for three ranges of standards for the 12 common proteins of serum. Three different standards with low, normal, and elevated values would be very useful in the clinical laboratory.

DR. KEITGES: Dr. Nakamura and I are working with the Diagnostic Immunology Resource Committee, helping in the development of the secondary standard for the CAP.

DR. HURTUBISE: Dr. Keitges, what units are going to be used for our baseline? What are we going to propose that people should use?

DR. NAKAMURA: That is a very good question, and one which remains unanswered at this point. I would like to propose the appointment of a task force. In addition, the CAP will make available control sera for the 12 proteins of normal, high, and low values based on ranges of clinical relevance of that particular protein. Considering the state of the art, I would propose that serum rather than plasma be used.

We considered plasma because some investigators wish to have control plasma with preservation of functional activity of complement. Serum standards for C3 have the problem of the C3 and the split products of C3. The problem with split products of C3 is not as evident in nephelometric assays as in radioimmunodiffusion assays. However, the standard should be good enough so that it can be used for radioimmunodiffusion assays as well as for other methods.

As far as assigning the gravimetric units, the primary and reference standard material must be agreed upon by the task force.

DR. KEITGES: Let us hope that we are more successful than the group that was trying to resolve the temperature for enzyme determinations.

DR. CAVALLARO: Has thought been given to abnormal standards? Often when we work with normal standards in the development of a procedure, it will work fine with those "normals," but when you encounter abnormal serum, for example a myeloma, there are proteins in myelomas that are not normally seen in "normal" standards. How would this affect the so-called standard procedure if we standardize on the normal?

DR. NAKAMURA: It is difficult to have normal and abnormal types of immunoglobulin standards since there are many different types of monoclonal proteins. Perhaps we can address ourselves to this problem in a resource committee with a proficiency survey sample. An abnormal sera with a high monoclonal protein can be sent, and a diversity of results can be expected depending upon the standard material and antisera used for quantitation.

QUESTION FROM THE FLOOR: We have always proposed that abnormal protein not be measured by quantitation as a general rule; if a patient with a monoclonal protein is being followed, the technique of electrophoresis should be employed.

DR. KEITGES: I'd like to turn the meeting over now to Dr. Bowman, chairman of the group on immunoenzyme assays.

IMMUNOENZYME ASSAYS

DR. BOWMAN: When the four chairmen met this morning, we went over the goals and discussed what the recommendations might be. You have already heard Dr. Keitges list the goals and recommendations; we then reviewed the consensus of opinion expressed by the members of our group. It was interesting that the same concepts and recommendations were unanimously agreed upon by our members. However, the semantics were different.

I'd like to read certain recommendations from the section on immunoenzyme assays. (1) By some priority system, standard control sera, characterized in several laboratories, must be made available for each test system. The priorities can probably be established by those tests which are presently being introduced into the routine diagnostic laboratories. (2) Standardization of reference and assay procedures is a primary need. (3) The advisability of investigation by a task force that each reagent for reference methods have a procedure for standardization was mentioned, but it was not the consensus of the group. We do not have a specific recommendation in our group and I think that this is the state of the art as we pointed out, by the very nature of the discussion, with the exception of the specific methodology which was presented by Dr. Schneider.

DR. WALLS: My main objectives are: standardization and obtaining accurate results by good techniques. Our group believes that many manufacturers also need such a good system. I think that this is a dilemma that has to be resolved eventually.

DR. SCHNEIDER: A comment made by Dr. Keitges regarding enzymeimmunology assay brings to mind that there has been a problem with semantics. Terminology needs standardization; the lack of it in the past has resulted in confusion.

DR. KEITGES: I'd like to turn the meeting over now to the chairman of the immunofluorescence group.

IMMUNOFLUORESCENCE

DR. NAKAMURA: Should fluorescent immunoassay be adopted as the official term? The state of the art is such that we can only come up with specific recommendations for the tissue assays.

Dr. Palmer's recommendations for quality control standardization in immunofluorescence assays are: (1) We select from the ample existing information pertinent to all aspects of immunofluorescence, the most appropriate procedural approach in established standardized methodology. (2) We should involve the commercial producers much more intimately in efforts to establish and proliferate the standardized methodology referred to in number one. (3) We continue efforts to make reference reagents available as standards along with the various immunofluorescence systems so that the first and second recommendations can be facilitated.

Dr. Horan feels that the application of cell sorters for routine clinical immunology testing is in the process of development as a method of the future. Immunochemical reagents are important for flow cytometry. The ideal fluorescent labeled reagent may be a monoclonal antibody fragment derived from antibody prepared in vitro with use of the hybridoma technique.

Specific recommendations which should be brought up for consideration to the group were presented by Dr. Beutner for tissue immunofluorescence assays. A specific recommendation for the tissue fluorescence assay is: A reference control serum for the indirect IF ANA test. Sera from three systemic lupus erythematosus patients, or those with other systemic rheumatic diseases, in which the specific number of antibodies has been characterized and identified by the other specific immunologic tests should be made available. The three proposed reagents would be: (1) A titer of 1:160 or greater in the indirect IF ANA test. (2) A titer in the borderline range of 20-80. (3) A normal sera in the range of less than 10 in the indirect IF ANA.

Which of the assay systems we are going to recommend is a problem to be considered by the task force. What type of assay procedures should one use to determine the titers of the control sera?

DR. BEUTNER: The suggestion was that the initial assays be done by two methods. One is the young rat liver section, the other is the mouse kidney section. The specific nuclear antigens would be assayed by conventional methods. They include double stranded DNA, Sm, RNP, and other antibodies.

Dr. Nakamura suggested that sera be made available from clinically documented cases of systemic lupus erythematosus having a titer of 160 or greater by the IF ANA mouse kidney assay. The second serum would be in the borderline range and the third serum would be in the negative-normal range. I feel that this type of SLE serum is of great fundamental importance because we need to understand clearly that there are cases of clinically difficult SLE that are ANA negative. I feel that it should be done by as many tests as possible to satisfy all concerned, that there is, indeed, such an SLE serum.

DR. NAKAMURA: The second recommendation by Dr. Beutner is the development of a low-cost device for assessing the sensitivity of the fluorescent optical system. An example of this would be microscopic slides with droplets and a carrier with particles carrying known quantitative amounts of fluorescence. The third recommendation is to draft quality control procedures for the indirect or the direct immunofluorescent test studies on biopsies and tissue procedures.

I would like to recommend the drafting of some kind of quality control procedures. One would like to stay away from the rigidly standardized methods because different methods can be acceptable if one has (1) determined normal values, (2) has established clinical relevance, and (3) can help the clinician in interpretation of the results. There are certain quality control procedures used in tissue immunofluorescent tests, for example, the use of a high and low titer pool and of sera to check each reagent. Also, a positive and negative control should be included in each run of patient samples. In the case of organ specific autoantibodies, one should include another section of tissue such as liver or kidney to test for non-specific immunofluorescence.

There are certain procedures that each laboratory should adopt to make certain that the results reported are accurate. Using the indirect IF ANA, many are attempting to establish a diagnosis with the test. A good sensitive test would be of help in ruling against the diagnosis of SLE when the indirect IF test is negative. In certain diseases, such as scleroderma, Sjögren's syndrome, 40% of the patients may show a negative immunofluorescent ANA test by the standard procedure. In these diseases, one can have a specific nuclear antibody which can be determined by other methods.

Probably one of the good substrates today for immunofluorescence testing would be one of the human B lymphocytes line that has an EB virus incorporated into the genome.

The only problem with using a cell line such as Wil$_2$ for an immunofluorescence test is that the desired nuclear antigen may be soluble and may be lost from the cell. Each cell bath should be checked for the presence of the nuclear antigens.

We should not limit the control sera to these two SLE sera, since in certain systemic rheumatic diseases, one cannot use IF ANA as a screening test because the patient may still demonstrate a specific nuclear antibody demonstrated by other specific tests.

Let's open this for discussion as to whether we want, as a group, to make a specific recommendation for providing some control sera for tissue immunofluorescence analysis, specifically indirect IF ANA test.

DR. NAKANE: In principle, I agree with Dr. Beutner. However, I feel that in this day and age, there are still many technical difficulties accompanying the recommendations made by Dr. Beutner. If one is just going to use IF ANA, it may be different. However, I'm sure he's not willing to stop with the ANA test. Control sera are not available in large quantities, and it would be difficult to adopt all of Dr. Beutner's recommendations.

DR. NAKAMURA: I believe Dr. Nakane is correct. It is difficult with the current state of the art in the United States to obtain a large amount of patient material for control sera. However, Dr. Beutner has a large source from the U.S. and foreign countries and he is able to actually make these reference control sera available. It would be difficult to obtain positive control sera in uncommon diseases such as hypoadrenalism. Dr. Beutner may be one of the few people who is able to obtain significant amounts of control sera. If significant amounts of borderline and positive sera are obtained, one can characterize it for presence of specific nuclear antibodies and supply each laboratory with 1ml. The individual laboratories could make dilutions and use the control serum as a reference material.

DR. RITCHIE: I disagree; I think the material is available in this country. I suppose it depends on the part of the country in which you are located, but cooperation from the public is to be expected. We've not had a great deal of difficulty in getting units of blood from individuals in the community once the need for it has been logically explained. I am anxious about taking material from overseas sources. It cannot be brought into the country legally.

DR. BEUTNER: I am in complete agreement with Dr. Nakane that we cannot do this for a great array of test systems in immunofluorescence. It is, however, possible to do it with the IF ANA test. This has a technical advantage in that, basically, the test systems we use for a fairly sizable group of immunofluorescent tests are completely comparable. Thus, if we are able to achieve reproducibility with one immunofluorescent test system, the prognosis becomes somewhat better for others. This is a step, but it is not a complete answer. It would be better to complete a workup on ANA and to then go into other types of test systems because the needs are so many that it is best to cover a broader field in the short time we have in our lives.

I agree with Dr. Ritchie that it is highly desirable to obtain materials from the United States. We are making vigorous efforts, and we have some liter quantities of the materials from the United States. We will continue to move in this direction—not using materials only from overseas—but this is where we are starting. This has all been cleared legally through customs; there are no secrets. Customs is concerned only with the infectious nature of the material, and this material is not infectious. We have consent forms from each of the donors stating that this material may be used for standardization of tests. This is the primary objective of the International Service for Immunological Laboratories, Inc. (ISIL), which is the sponsoring organization for making these volume reference sera available.

DR. HURTUBISE: I would like to make a comment regarding the conjugate and its specificity. As one deals with the Fiax assay, which is fluorescent immunoassay, the type of reagents used in these assays has tremendous application in the cellular immune assays, including B and T-cell analyses. It has some application in terms of defining the specificities of the conjugates; fluorescence is the test with the most sensitivity, and perhaps as a standard it should be used to define specificity; perhaps the fluorescent beads are of technical value.

DR. NAKAMURA: It is my impression from this discussion that these controls should be made available and we should make an effort to obtain the sera from donors in the United States. Many of us have had difficulty in finding cooperative clinicians and patients to collect significant amounts of positive control sera.

DR. KEITGES: I want to reemphasize and underscore a recommendation that has already been mentioned. Rather than addressing ourselves to a reference immunofluorescent method, we should address ourselves to specific recommendations for quality control of existing methods.

DR. NAKAMURA: I would recommend that we form some task force which would establish certain quality control procedures which would be applicable to various common methods.

DR. HORAN: The cell sorter may be helpful in tissue fluorescence immunoassays. Since it is a non-subjective measure, it may be helpful in determining the intensities of titers of various sera. By using standard single cell suspension such as tissue culture lines, one is able to actually measure the fluorescence intensity, or each cell line, and determine titers with an objective measure.

DR. BEUTNER: This certainly has great value in studies of B-cells and other systems in which one deals with a surface antigen.

The performance of tests on ANA with a viable cell suspension is not possible because the ANA fails to react with the nuclei; they do not penetrate the intact cell. Certainly the cell sorter is a powerful tool in certain areas, but not in others.

DR. NAKAMURA: This was specifically addressed in the second recommendation concerning the optical device to calibrate quantitation of fluorescence.

DR. HORAN: It is also possible to look at ANA using a flow cytometer. We do it with fixed cells, and in that case, the antibody penetrates very nicely. If cells are fixed in suspension, it is easy to make an objective measurement from any internal antigen. One has to be concerned about the loss of antigen, although we see the same patterns, speckled, rimmed, etc., even after the cells are fixed.

DR. NAKAMURA: You are correct. We fix the cells so the cellular antigens do not leach out, but certain of the antigens, such as the rheumatoid arthritis or rheumatoid associated nuclear antigens, may be denatured with fixation.

DR. KEITGES: I'd now like to turn the meeting over to Dr. Deodhar, chairman of the cell-mediated immunity group.

DR. DEODHAR: In the area of cellular immunology or cell-mediated immunity, in order to remain consistent with the rest of the terminology, we should call the procedures cellular immunoassays. In this group, there were certain points upon which there was a definite consensus. First of all, we agreed that the state of the art in this area was such that no one procedure could be enshrined as the definitive procedure for the purpose of developing quality control or standards. We would advise a cautious period of waiting until we have a better idea of which of the procedures are valid, which of them have definite clinical relevance. At the present time, we do not feel that it is advisable to recommend any one procedure in terms of quality controls or developing standards. However, we do feel that some sort of checklist should be developed for the purpose of providing guidelines to laboratories that are interested in performing assays of this type. Perhaps the CAP Diagnostic Immunology Resource Committee would be the group to develop this type of checklist.

Another area in which there was also general agreement, except for a few instances such as in lymphoproliferative diseases and immune deficiency diseases, was that of the cellular immunoassays which do not provide a diagnostic test, but rather are tests that are helpful in understanding the genesis and natural history of a given disease. We should look at these procedures from that standpoint. Another recommendation was that perhaps a task force could be developed to provide some type of standard cell preparation. I am thinking of perhaps a frozen lymphocyte preparation which could be used for providing different laboratories with some kind of material that has been pretested in various experienced laboratories.

This is really the only specific recommendation we can make at this point. Basically, we all agreed with Dr. Rose's comment that this is perhaps a time for cautious waiting so that some of the test procedures which are not going to stand up to the test of time will eventually die their own death.

DR. BARNA: Some of my comments may be a bit naive, but considering the type of assay that we are talking about, I think our whole concept may change. Until now it was very easy to say, "Here is humoral immunity; that's antibody. Ah! Here's cellular immunity; those are cells." As we can see now, cellular immunity involves humoral immunity; it's the soluble factors. It appears to me that we may well end up dividing what we now call cellular immunity into a series of assays that simply look at cells and membranes, look at soluble factors, and really look at cell functions such as phagocytosis. Perhaps in this cautious waiting period, we'll discover that some of these assays may never be useful.

DR. DEODHAR: This is one point that Dr. Yoshida also emphasizes, that perhaps in the future we may be doing assays, whether they are radioimmunoassays or fluorescent immunoassays, with respect to some of the non-specific factors involved in cellular immune mechanisms.

DR. YOSHIDA: The chairman mentioned the checklist point for the future, but we must recognize that in some of the basic procedures, such as mitogen stimulation or migration inhibition assays, many laboratories are already using a checklist for the procedures. In addition to the checklist, we should try to point out the major points of variation in these assays. Technically, some of these cellular immune assays have many variations in procedure. We are approaching the point where some type of standardization of each "major" assay is possible and should be made.

DR. DEODHAR: I think these are questions which are best answered through the task force approach. We are only now ready to deal with specifics.

DR. HURTUBISE: Having done many of these assays on a clinical basis at the request of physicians, I have found that there is a priority list that can be generated in terms of examining some of the techniques. It is obvious to me that the assay which is closest to applying some standards would be the B and T-cell assays. We are beginning to get many requests from small laboratories as to how the assays are performed. I think a checklist for the procedure would be very appropriate.

The area of lymphoblastic transformation in the lymphocytic tests becomes very confusing. Dr. Rose indicated the problem of expressing results in stimulation index versus counts per minute. I think we have a huge problem in this area, even in the basic biology of the responsive lymphocytes. Are we really measuring the right component, DNA synthesis? Should we be measuring protein synthesis?

Should we be measuring lipid turnover and a variety of other things at least in terms of their clinical relevance? There has been some effort toward standardization of the lymphoblastic transformation tests; there is a recent article in *Cancer Research* by Dr. Herbermann's group in which they indicate that each time a transformation test is done, they compare daily a pool of cells and look at the stimulation index of that pool. One can compare the variability of the culture, isotope, and counter.

This is a valuable step in the direction of quality control. The third level of priority would be looking at the areas of lymphokine production. I am sure that Dr. Yoshida will agree with me that MIF is not a good assay for the laboratory.

I do think the standardization B and T-cell assay is approachable at this particular stage. The reagents should be defined.

Our past experience with compiling data when doing cellular immunology assays has been that accurate clinical records must be kept if the assays are to have clinical relevance.

DR. KEITGES: We have found an effective way of dealing with that situation at our institution. We request that before those tests are done, we are brought into consultation on the case in question; we then are personally involved in the patient's care, and we may enter into the clinical record.

DR. HORAN: Much of the work in cellular immunology has been done in human systems and we would really like more research. This body of the CAP could help influence national councils in an attempt to direct some money toward research; this would result in a better understanding of the assays for cellular immunology. We must have a very good understanding and basic knowledge of the mechanisms operating at the cellular level of these assays. Until then, the value of these assays in the clinical setting is going to be diminished.

DR. DEODHAR: It is very difficult to obtain funds for studies of this type. However, with the cooperative effort of the CAP and organizations other than the NIH, we may be more successful.

DR. CHANDOR: Dr. Hurtubise and others have stated that some education and guidance should be given to the clinician in areas of autoimmune antibody studies and cellular immunology assays. Some clinicians have ordered anti-DNA studies without ever doing an ANA. We get many requests for B and T-cells only to discover that the patient has been on chemotherapy and the white count is 1,000. Skin tests are not done prior to requests for cell transformation. There are many things that the task force could adapt as guidelines for laboratories if they want to teach clinicians how to use these tests. We find this to be very important, especially in the area of B and T-cell transformation. I think that if a conference such as this recommended that education become an integral part of quality control, one would see a change and better utilization of these procedures.

DR. NAKAMURA: We have a general clinical research center laboratory at our institution in which cellular immune assays are performed. We use various researchers' procedures and try to adapt the procedures to human patients. There are certain criteria for establishment of the assays for accurate reproducible performances. For example, recovery studies for the procedure on isolation of lymphocytes should be done. Normal values should be determined along with the clinical relevance so that one can interpret the results.

I would like to see the task force address itself to a detailed checklist for a certain procedure.

My last comment is that there should be some leadership in the task force which should not be concerned only with methodology since methods will change. We want to reach the right answer to the question of the particular disease problem. The task force should determine the current state of the art as to what testing we recommend, and what other procedures should be considered to answer "clinical relevance."

DR. KEITGES: We're going to have to select specific target areas for task force activity. I know most of the groups involved. The CAP certainly has a commitment that any standards it develops will go through the NCCLS consensus mechanism, and I know the NCCLS will be more than happy to lend its aid to this task force approach. We've talked about liaison with international bodies so there will be no duplication.

DR. NAKAMURA: The task force concept is great. How about funding?

DR. KEITGES: Much depends on the manner in which it is set up. I could see that the DIRC may want to take on a certain project, so this would fall under the auspices of the CAP. I can see the NCCLS wanting to take on a certain project, so this would then be its problem. We may go to some group, perhaps an international body. I do not have the answer to all of it. We may find a task force and have to find somebody to support its activity. Funding of this operation as far as the CAP is concerned ends today with the Conference, but that does not mean that they "wash their hands of it." They will long be interested in the proceedings and any projects that the DIRC decides to take on. Logically, I think they would incorporate the expertise in this room.

First I would designate where we think the task force activity is needed and also, perhaps, the personnel. Then the next step—would funding be a CAP function or an outside function, or just who would fund it? One will never find a more effective tool than this task force approach. I've seen a task force of nine or ten dedicated people volunteering their time on weekends, meeting five or six times, and accomplishing what you might have thought would take years to do.

I continue to stress clinical relevance; expending precious time and precious funds on an exercise that either is academic or a futility is grossly inappropriate when resources are so drastically limited.

I feel that this has been a most outstanding and successful conference. I want to thank all areas of government, industry, and professional groups for your contribution.

INDEX

B-5 fluorescein filters 117
B-galactosidase 67, 118
B-galactosyl umbelliferone 118
B-galactosyl umbelliferone-gentamicin 118
Bienenstock 28
bilirubin 147
Binder, W.L. 89
binding sites 14
biological false positive 142
biuret method 94
blastogenic response 105
blast transformation 135
blood 3
Borgen 28
Bowman 164
Boyden 10
bromide 39
buffer 3
Buffone 14, 26, 28
BUN 177
Burtin 10
BV type filters 92

C

C$_3$ 11
C$_4$ 19
^{14}C 49
caffeine 55
Caslake 29
Cambiaso 28
candida 127
candida antigen (dermatophyton) 143
canine heart worm 158
carbonara 10
carcinogen 82
catalase 75
Cawley, Leo P. 1
CEA 155
cell-mediated immunity 126, 174
cellular immunology 173
Center for Disease Control candidate preparation number 3 149, 159
centrifugal analyzer 15
Chagas' disease 81
chemiluminescence 50
chemotactic 126
chemotactic assays 135
chemotaxis 128
chessboard titrations 92
chloride 39

8-chlorotheophylline 55
cholesterol 159
Chromium-51 128
Chromium-51 labeled cells 128
chromogen 80
chromophoric hapten 112
chronic granulomatous diseases 176
chronic lymphocytic leukemia 134
Clarke 10
Clem 83
^{14}C-leucine 136
Cleveland Clinic Foundation Department of Immunopathology 126
CMV 90
colchicine 108
Cole 177
College of American Pathologists 159
College of American Pathologists Diagnostic Immunology Resource Committee 164
colorimeters 64
complement 6, 90
complement (C3) 29
complement fixation 64
complement fixation antigen 81
complement 1Q (C1Q) 75
complement receptors 105, 144
computer 15
concanavalin A 127
conjugate 90, 156, 161
continuous flow systems 11
control sera 167
Cooke polystyrene (PS) 80
Cooke polyvinyl chloride (PVC) 80
corticosteroid 98
counterelectrophoresis 3
CPK isoenzyme 7
C-reactive protein 20
Creveling 27
cross-reactions 142
cuvette 15
cysteine 76
cytochrome C 76
cytophilic antibody 132
cytotoxic assays 135
cytotoxic drugs 127

D

Daigneault 27, 29
Daniels 173
Datiles 26

incident light 11
incubation 82
indirect cell-bound virus EIAs 67
indirect IF tests 90
infectious disease 126
in-liquid continuous flow immunoanalysis 24
interference 13
interferon 144
International Federation of Clinical Chemistry 32
International Service for Immunology Laboratories
  (ISIL) 91, 165
International Union of Immunological Societies (IUIS)
  82, 91, 149
International Units 32, 150
iodothyronine 112
ionic strength 14
ions 14
3-isobutyl-1-methylxanthine 55
isoenzymes 7
isotope 2
IUSIS 168

J

Jerne hemolytic plaque assays 157

K

Kabakoff, D.S. 47
Kabat 10
kappa 6
karyotyping 108
Keitges, Pierre W. 162
Kendall 10
Keren 26
Killingsworth, L.M. 11, 26, 31
Kirby-Bauer 168
kits 10
Kumar, V. 89
Kusnetz 26

L

labeled antigen 48
lactic dehydrogenase 159
LAI phenomenon 132
lambda 6
laser-nephelometer 27
latex-coated beads 80
latex particles 28
Laurell 3, 10
Leinikii 80, 84
Lemieux 27

Leone 11
leukemia 56
leukemia virus 158
leukocyte adherence inhibition assay (LIA) 132
Li 11
light chains 147, 169
light-scattering 11
light-scattering analysis 26
light-scatter intensity 105
Linbro polystyrene 80
lipemia 147
lipopolysaccharide 127
liposomes 117, 158
liquid chromatography 176
liquid N_2 92
L-lysine 76
Lou 10
low-density lipoproteins 29
luminol derivatives 50
lupus band test 162
lymphocyte mitogenic factor 144
lymphocytes 103, 174
lymphocyte transformation 134
lymphokines 126, 135, 176
lymphoproliferative disease 127
lymphotoxins 135, 144
lysozyme 28

M

macrophage 126, 174
macrophage activation 135
macrophage migration inhibition (MMI) 133
malate dehydrogenase 51
malignancy 126
Mancini 10
Mansberg 26
Masson 28
mass units 32
maximum reaction rate 37
Maxwell 27
McKelvey 10
measles-infected epithelial cells 127
Meloy 95
methotrexate 56
1-methyl-xanthine 55
Michelle-Dutton type cultures 104
microELISA 80
microperoxidase 76
microscopy 17
microtitration plates 80

polystyrene microcuvettes 80
polystyrene microspheres 105, 106
polystyrene tubes 80
polyvalent conjugate 92
polyvinyl microtitration 67
porcine esterase 119
positive controls 161
post-transplant hepatic disease 134
PPD 127, 143
precipitin curve 12, 34
precipitin zone 3
primary standards 20
protease inhibitors 32
protein 6
protein-bound iodine 59
psoriasis 56
Putnam 24

Q

quartz halogen 92
quartz plate 114
quartz-water interface 114
Quash 28
quenching 50, 115

R

rabbit anti-human IgG 117
radialimmunodiffusion (RID) 2
radiation 13
radioimmunoassay (RIA) 7, 49, 60
radiolabeled thymidine 127
radionuclides 49
Ramslo 28
Rayleigh's law 12
reactant-labeled methods 61
reaction rate 37
reagents 148
red cell receptors 105
Reeves 10
reference sera 90
reference standard 90
Reijngoad 28
Reimer, Charles 24
Ressler 3
reverse competitive electroimmunodiffusion (RC EID) 7
reverse single gel diffusion 2
rheumatoid factor 107
rheumatology 176
rhodamine 103

RhoGAM 107
Rh positive fetal cells 107
Riccomi 28
Ritchie, Robert 11, 23, 24, 26, 27, 29
Roch 28
Rose, Noel R. 141, 173
rosettes 127
rubella 155
Ruitenberg 80

S

saline 11, 38
salting out 40
sandwich technique 115
sarcoidosis 127
Saunders, George C. 63, 158
Savory, John 9, 11, 26
scattergram 57
Scheidegger 10
Schneider, Richard 47, 168
Schram 28
Schultze 11
Schwick 11
scleroderma 170
Sieber 27
semi-automated dilutor 17
sensitivity 5, 38, 43
Sephadex beads 80
Sephadex G-100 135
serum glutamic oxaloacetic transaminase (SGOT) 113
serum protein 5
Sezary syndrome 134
Shanbron 10
Shapiro 29
sheep erythrocytes 103
sheep red blood cells (E) 127
signal-to-noise ratio 17
simple gel diffusion test 96
Sjögren's syndrome 170
skin test antigens 143
SK/SD 143
SLE 98, 162
Smith, L. 29
Smith, R.S. 27
sodium chloride 14
sodium fluoride 39
solid phase antigen 113
solid phase enzyme immunoassays 64
solid phase immunoadsorbent 28
solid phase matrix 85

Sommers 168
specificity 43
spectrophotofluorometer 15
spectrophotometer 11
spinal fluid 3
spleen 144
standard deviations 38
standard reagents 161
Sternberg, J.C. 27
steroids 127
Stevens 28
substrate 51
syphilis 117, 170
Syva Company 49

T

T_3 155
T_4 59, 155
Tager 28
target cells 137
T-cell 103, 127, 174
T-cell antiserum 127
$T\mu$ cells 175
$T\gamma$ cells 175
temperature 14, 82
tetraethyl rhodamine 116
tetrahydrocannabinol (THC) 51
tetramethyl 116
T-helper lymphocytes 175
theobromine 54
theophylline 54
therapeutic control agents (TCA) 52
thymosin 176
thyroid 58, 155
thyroxine (T_4) 58, 112
Tiffany 15
tissue immunofluorescence 163
tissue phase 162
titer 35, 170
tonsils 144
Toxoplasma gondii 90
TPS-1 cell sorter 108
transferrin 11, 29
transplantation 126
transport proteins 32
tricophyton 143
tris-chloride buffer 38
tritiated proline 128
tritiated thymidine 105
trypsin 76

T-suppressor lymphocytes 175
tumor immunology 173
tungsten-halogen lamp 16
tungsten/iodine light source 15
T_3 uptake 155
T_4 uptake 155
turbidimetric analysis 11
Tween 20 68
Tween 80 68
two-dimensional IEP 4
two-dimensional titration 92
two-parameter cell sorter 106
Type III pneumococcus polysaccharide 10

U

ultraviolet spectroscopic analysis 16
urea 14
urine 3
UV type filters 92

V

Vaerman 28
Virella 27, 28
viruses 65
visible spectroscopic analysis 16
Voller 80

W

Walker 29
Walls, Kenneth 79, 155, 161
wavelength 13, 112
Wegfahrt 11
white count differential 176
Williams 10, 11
Williamson 29
World Health Organization (WHO) 81, 156

X

xanthines 55
Xenon 92

Y

Yolken 83
Yoshida, Takeshi 131, 176
Young 27

Z

zone electrophoresis 20
zone of growth inhibition 169